Take Care

Take Care

A Memoir of Love, Family and Never Giving Up

Lindsey
Burrow

with Donald McRae

C

CENTURY

CENTURY

UK | USA | Canada | Ireland | Australia
India | New Zealand | South Africa

Century is part of the Penguin Random House group of companies
whose addresses can be found at global.penguinrandomhouse.com

Penguin Random House UK,
One Embassy Gardens, 8 Viaduct Gardens, London SW11 7BW

penguin.co.uk

Penguin
Random House
UK

First published 2025
001

Copyright © Lindsey Burrow, 2025

Set in 11.5/17.7pt Sabon LT Std
Typeset by Jouve (UK), Milton Keynes

Printed and bound in Great Britain by Clays Ltd, Elcograf S.p.A.

The authorised representative in the EEA is Penguin Random House Ireland,
Morrison Chambers, 32 Nassau Street, Dublin D02 YH68

A CIP catalogue record for this book is available from the British Library

ISBN: 978-1-529-94133-3

Penguin Random House is committed to a sustainable future
for our business, our readers and our planet. This book is made
from Forest Stewardship Council® certified paper.

MIX
Paper | Supporting
responsible forestry
FSC
www.fsc.org   FSC® C018179

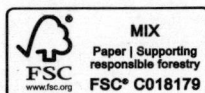

For Macy, Maya and Jackson – love lives forever x

In loving memory of my husband, Rob,
who continues to inspire me every day.

Contents

Foreword by HRH Prince William

Like many people, I became aware of Rob Burrow's heart-breaking diagnosis with motor neurone disease through the incredible fundraising efforts being carried out by Rob and his loved ones, including his friend and former teammate Kevin Sinfield. The phenomenal support given to this legend of the rugby league world was powerful and moving to witness.

I was delighted when Rob and Kevin were awarded their CBEs at the end of 2023, in recognition of their raising £15 million and invaluable levels of awareness to help fight such a terrible disease. I was so honoured to go to Leeds to present their honours in a place that meant so much to both of them: Headingley Stadium.

During that visit, the love and admiration for Rob and all that he had achieved – both on and off the pitch – was evident. Although after hearing about the pranks he used to play on his teammates, I'm sure there were moments when his targets might have had a few choice words to say about him!

Despite the advanced nature of Rob's condition, I was struck by the incredible strength, positivity and resilience of Lindsey.

Rob told me that Lindsey was far tougher than any of the men he had played with, or against, over the years. I know that I am not alone in feeling great admiration for how she has kept going in the face of such adversity.

Coming to terms with such a horrific diagnosis, delivered at a time when the family were looking forward to the next chapter of their lives following Rob's retirement, must have been almost too much to bear.

Lindsey's unwavering love for and dedication to her husband has been plain to see, both throughout his illness and following his tragic passing. Her immediate response to the devastating news of Rob's diagnosis was to do everything she could to look after and support him, eventually providing round-the-clock care and tending to his every need.

Alongside this she continued to work while raising their three young children and, crucially, supporting them to understand and process such difficult and life-changing news.

Those caring for family members themselves shoulder unimaginable burdens. Their selflessness, kindness and compassion for others dramatically reduces pressure on our services, but the work they carry out is often behind closed doors and therefore sadly under-recognised.

Throughout Rob's illness, the family's openness about their experiences will have helped countless others, not only through raising the profile of MND and the funds to fight it, but also by helping those going through similar situations to know that they are not alone.

These pages contain Lindsey's story of compassion, perseverance and love. By sharing her story, she is shining a light on those who are dealing with incredibly difficult situations, putting others' needs before their own, and making great personal sacrifices every day.

I hope this book provides all those going through their own challenges with some comfort and optimism, and that it inspires us all to look out for one another.

Prologue
The Last Goodbye

Sunday 7 July 2024, Pontefract

The hearse, which carries my husband Rob, is due to arrive in fifteen minutes. The children and I are ready and waiting in the front room at twelve-thirty. My mum and dad and my brother, Mark, as well as Rob's parents and sisters, are with us. We will fill the two big black cars that follow the hearse at the head of the cortege. This is an excruciating time and the wait feels endless. Macy, Maya and Jackson are already upset and I'm trying hard to hold us all together.

Lesley, the humanist celebrant we have chosen to lead the service, has been attentive and thoughtful. She has visited our family twice to hear our memories of Rob as well as our wishes for the funeral. I knew we had made the right choice when Lesley said it sounded to her as if the funeral should be a celebration of how Rob lived, rather than a lamentation of how he died. This is exactly what we need now.

But I am still anxious and can't quite fulfil Rob's example of living in the moment. I desperately want the service to go well and to do justice to Rob. Most of all, I am worried about the children and how they might be affected. Macy is twelve, Maya is nine and Jackson is just five. They have never been to a funeral before: when my Nana Nancy died in 2020, we couldn't attend because of Covid.

We took the kids to the crematorium yesterday afternoon. It felt important to show them what to expect and to give the girls a chance to practise their short eulogies. Macy and Maya are determined to read the words I've helped them write for their dad. But I'm afraid the enormity of the occasion, and our grief, might be too much for them as they will be the first two speakers.

I slept terribly knowing that we are about to say our final goodbye to Rob.

At last the undertakers, a few minutes early, drive up our little road and slow to a stop outside the front door. I go out to meet them and Eddie, the senior funeral director, is sombre but lovely. He makes sure that we are ready but moves very slowly. I just want to get going but Eddie is almost ninety and there is no rushing him.

Before we climb into the cars Eddie suggests that he could walk ahead of the cortege for some of the route – perhaps both at the start and then at the end of the two-and-a-half-mile journey to the crematorium. It is a kind gesture because it would add to the dignified solemnity of the occasion (although I privately wonder if we will ever get there if a walking Eddie leads the way). But the more serious thought is that extending the agony for the children will be almost unbearable. As tactfully as I can, I suggest to Eddie that it would be best if we just get there as the funeral is meant to start at 1pm. He nods and suggests that he will save his walk for the moment when we enter the grounds of the crematorium on Wakefield Road.

'Thank you, Eddie,' I say as I usher the children into the lead car with Rob's mum and dad, Irene and Geoff. Mark and my parents, Sharon and Graham, and Rob's two sisters, Joanne and Claire, climb into the second car.

Macy and Maya look drawn and pale, while Jackson is just uncertain. He clutches the worry worm that the nurses gave him the night before we lost Rob. It was a strangely beautiful night, with the children showing Rob such love. He had been in the grip of motor neurone disease for four and a half years and he couldn't talk or move. Trapped in his ravaged body, totally paralysed and at a point where he could hardly swallow while also struggling to breathe, Rob was a ghostly shadow of the man he had once been. At just five foot five, Rob had been a giant of rugby league and a key member of the brilliant Leeds Rhinos team, which dominated the game for many years. His teammates rallied round him, and Barrie McDermott and Kevin Sinfield visited him in hospital in his final days, while admitting that they had been blown away by Rob's positivity and courage throughout his long battle with MND.

Rob's character is so evident in our children and, moving beyond the profound sadness of his last night alive, Macy, Maya and Jackson were brave and uplifting. They had painted their dad's fragile fingers so that they could make prints for our memory box and he had watched, drowsy with morphine, as they held his hands with such care. The last photograph I ever took of Rob captures him smiling in his hospital bed, surrounded by love and our three children.

Our memories of that night sustain us now. Each of the children received a little knitted worm from the hospital staff, and Jackson takes so much comfort from this gift. It's almost as if his worry worm will protect him because he now won't leave home without it. Although it looks a little threadbare after five weeks, his worry worm retains its magical powers. Jackson holds it tightly now as he looks calmly out of the window.

Maya always goes to bed with the knitted heart that she had placed in her dad's hands in hospital, and sleeps with it under her pillow every night. Macy, meanwhile, treasures the lock of her dad's hair that she had cut, so tenderly, before he slipped away. It is her most important keepsake.

For me, different memories help me through the pain. Of course the more recent images in my head are sometimes harrowing, as I cared for Rob for years when he could no longer feed himself or go to the toilet. But I loved him beyond measure. I had first gone out with Rob when we were fifteen and we'd lived together for more than half of our forty-one years of life. There are so many snapshots of our sunlit joy in my head. Even death cannot dent, let alone erase, my love for Rob.

The cortege crawls through Pontefract. We take nearly an hour, rather than the expected fifteen minutes, to make the short drive. The roads are thronged on either side by thousands of people who have come to pay their respects. They wear rugby shirts of all colours to show how much Rob means to everyone in the game. I am just as moved when I see elderly people and teenage girls and boys, as well as mothers and their children, waiting patiently for the hearse to pass. They do not look like rugby supporters – just ordinary people, spanning the generations, who want to say thank you and goodbye to Rob.

People step forward and touch the hearse, or leave flowers on its shiny black surface. Others stand and applaud with heartfelt warmth. I feel choked up, seeing all these people, as well as the respectful expressions on individual faces. I sometimes feel like I should wave in gratitude, but I don't want anyone to think we regard ourselves as famous or special.

We are as ordinary as everyone standing on these streets. We come from the same community and share the same history. Rob never forgot this simple truth. He was born in Pontefract, raised in Castleford (where he started playing rugby before his junior career flourished at Featherstone Lions) and then joined the Academy at Leeds. He was revered for so many of the twenty years he spent at the Rhinos, first as a player and then as a coach.

Since his public battle with MND, Rob has become far more famous for a deeper cause. There have been so many tributes to his strength and humour and the way he raised awareness of MND as well as many millions of pounds to help fight the disease. In the wake of his death on 2 June 2024, famous sportsmen and -women, actors and politicians, and tens of thousands of unknown people, took to social media to say that Rob had touched their lives.

Prince William posted a message on X: *A legend of Rugby League, Rob Burrow had a huge heart. He taught us, 'in a world full of adversity, we must dare to dream.' Catherine and I send our love to Lindsey, Jackson, Maya and Macy. W*

The prime minister, Rishi Sunak, went on X too: *Rob was an inspiration to everyone who met him or who heard his incredible story. I was honoured to spend some time with him last year. He drove a fundraising campaign that supports vital new research improving the care for others – not least through the creation of The Rob Burrow Centre for Motor Neurone Disease in Leeds. He leaves behind an amazing legacy and my thoughts are with his friends and family.*

Rob would have been amused, rather than boastful, that the prime minister was talking about him. He once said in an interview that Kevin Sinfield would make a far better prime minister than Boris Johnson (or Bo-Jo, as he called him). I wish I could hear the joke Rob would have dreamed up if he had known that, on the day he died, all the major party leaders echoed each other as they spoke about him. He would also have been amazed, while hiding his modesty behind a cheeky quip.

Keir Starmer, locked in an election battle and just a month away from becoming the new prime minister, wrote on X: *Extremely sad news. Rob leaves behind an incredible legacy in his work to raise awareness and advocate for those with Motor Neurone Disease. My thoughts are with his family and friends through this time.*

Many people had picked up on Kev Sinfield's generous words: 'Rob shows us how to live and Lindsey shows us how to love.'

I believe that we can all draw valuable lessons from Rob who, amid brutal suffering, still found light and laughter in life. Rob made the most of every minute he had left after he was diagnosed with MND and, rather than crying about his misfortune, he savoured his time with the children, me, all his family and his friends. And, instead of wailing about the horrors of his disease, he was the face of a campaign that has raised over £20 million for research into MND, while helping the world understand what the illness meant.

So I endorsed Kev, absolutely, in believing that Rob taught us the importance of setting aside our – often trivial – daily worries, our insecurities and jealousies, while concentrating on all that truly matters in life. As Rob always said, when he could still talk, 'Life is for living.' It didn't matter to him that he was doubted or tested. When he was dismissed as being too small to play rugby and, later, when he was told at the outset of his diagnosis that he had just a year to live, Rob just tried harder and enjoyed as much of life as he could.

I had resolved to try and be a little more like Rob and draw on previously untapped reserves of courage and joy.

So while it meant a lot to be praised by Kev, and his words about me were humbling, I didn't feel I had done anything different to what almost anyone else would do in my situation. Who wouldn't want to care for the person they had loved for so many years? Who wouldn't do as much as they could to try and ease the agony of their husband or wife, son or daughter? I think we would all try to care compassionately for those we love most.

Rather than being remarkable, I believe that the care and love I showed to Rob was just an example of the same dedication and empathy that tens of thousands of people offer to loved ones who are facing illness, disability or a terminal disease every day. We are all the same, in trying our very best in arduous and draining situations. We all sometimes feel bereft and lonely, helpless and sad, as we battle against often impossible odds.

I'm well aware that I am so much more fortunate than most carers in this country. Rob's sporting renown gave us a platform where we could be showered with love and support, emotionally and financially, which few other families in similar circumstances would ever receive. The last years have been bruising for me, but I often wonder: how would I have coped without such help? I doubt that I could have matched the quiet and solitary heroism of all those carers who do just as much as I did – and more, without having the backing of the Leeds Rhinos, the BBC, the wider media and sporting worlds, and the unstinting support of the public.

Those unheralded carers deserve the plaudits far more than I do.

All these contrasting thoughts tumble through me in the car as we gaze at the sea of love for Rob. Twenty thousand people have turned out to line the streets. I remind the kids how their dad was admired and even adored.

But Macy speaks for all of us when, softly, she asks this question of Rob's illness and death: 'Why did it have to be my dad?'

There is no answer to such a raw question and so I try to explain how much their dad did for so many people. It's right to feel sad, but we should feel proud too.

Eventually, we turn in to the grounds of the crematorium. The summer rain has eased and watery sunshine makes the gardens glisten.

We step out of the car and I feel the eyes of our sixty guests drawn to me and the children. I lead them to the front entrance where Lesley smiles and takes my hand. I remind Macy, Maya and Jackson that we need to wait – we can only enter the crematorium after the pall-bearers have carried Rob to the altar.

A knot of anxiety twists in my gut. This is it. The moment of our final goodbye is almost here.

We see the coffin and the flowers and it suddenly hits us with fresh force. I gather all three of my children around me and hold them close. Despite this devastation we will find a way. We will go on together. I feel this so clearly. Even if we cry again about the loss of their cherished dad, and my beloved Rob, we won't let him down. We will try and make sure that, if he could look down on Pontefract now, Rob would feel so proud of us.

I

Shell Shock

Our lives will be blown apart today, but I feel the same old beautiful thrill as my train rumbles into Leeds. I know Rob will be waiting inside the station and, despite the worry of the past weeks, happiness ripples through me at the thought of seeing him.

We still feel young, at thirty-seven, and Rob has been my one and only love since we were fifteen. A month ago we moved our gorgeous family into our dream home. Life seems almost perfect.

The girls brim with life and creativity, showing such spark and ambition. Macy is eight years old and imagining a future where she plays the lead role in a musical theatre smash hit in the West End. Maya is still only four but she already fancies the idea of becoming a movie star. They laugh shyly whenever they tell me their grand plans because they know that all that really matters to their chatterbox of a mum is that they are happy and kind to everyone they meet.

My good mood is sealed by the fact that their little brother, our baby boy, Jackson, will turn one this Saturday. Our preparations for a special birthday party are in place and family and friends will make it a celebration to remember.

I know that Rob secretly dreams of Jackson following him and playing rugby league for Leeds Rhinos one day but, right now, my husband is more excited by the party. We believe that, before long, Rob will have the simple pleasure of passing a ball back and forth to his boy, before taking Jackson to a game when he is old enough to care about sport.

Rob, like me, just wants the kids to have joyful and fulfilled lives and so smiled when I once joked that I would like it more if Jackson became a ballet dancer. I've had enough dread to last me a lifetime after all the times I've been so concerned seeing Rob, at just five foot five, facing so many hulking giants and hard men.

The fact that Rob played almost 500 games for Leeds and won eight Super League Grand Finals and eighteen international caps helps me believe he is going to be okay. Of course I know he's not indestructible – I was there on that frightening day when he was knocked out badly in a World Cup match. The sight of Rob looking lifeless shook me to the core. I was also upset at all the other times he left the field with concussion or a broken collarbone.

But Rob was so tough, mentally and physically, that the brutal hits never fazed him. You need that resilience when you're up against men twice your size. Rob seemed fearless but, as a physiotherapist and his wife, I saw the impact on his body season after season.

It was a relief that he had played his last game, in a winning

Grand Final, two years earlier. There was another little dash of romance because, in that 2017 match at Old Trafford, Rob helped Leeds beat Castleford Tigers, the club that my family once supported so passionately. Pontefract, our home town, is just three miles from Castleford.

Leeds became our team, however, because of Rob. After his family and me, the Rhinos were the love of Rob's life. He joined their Academy in 1999 and spent the next eighteen years, and his entire professional career, at Leeds. Rob played alongside his great friends – amazing men including Barrie McDermott, Jamie Jones-Buchanan, Danny McGuire, Kevin Sinfield and Jamie Peacock.

Rugby league, like real life, is a harsh business. For all the titles and plaudits, Rob had his share of disappointments. In his final years, despite playing better than ever, he was often left on the bench by head coach Brian McDermott. He would come on and change the course of a match and, while the demand to start him grew louder, McDermott argued that his decision was vindicated because Rob always tore through the exhausted opposition with deadly effect.

Even his most unforgettable performance, in the 2011 Grand Final against St Helens, had been as a first-half substitute. The score was locked at 6–6, in a bruising game played in sheeting rain, when Rob came on earlier than usual. I normally watched quietly, willing Rob to just finish the match safely in one piece, but even I jumped up and screamed as he popped up like a jack-in-a-box, ran like a whippet and danced like a spinning top through the helpless Saints defence.

He received a pass just over the halfway line and the brilliance burst out of him. Rob stepped off his left foot and arrowed towards one of the big Saints forwards, before zipping around him. He avoided another heavy tackle, sidestepped their fullback Paul Wellens, putting him on his backside, and skipped past an attempted tap-tackle. Four defenders closed on him from various angles, but Rob flew towards the line and dived over.

It was one of the great Grand Final tries and he was swamped by his jubilant teammates, who could barely believe what he had just done. Rob's dancing feet and electric pace then set up Ryan Hall's try and, after Leeds cruised to victory, he was awarded the Harry Sunderland Trophy, for a second time, as Man of the Match.

He is a little superman. When he holds me close and tells me that everything will be all right, it's easy to believe him. I feel strangely sure that our visit to the specialist this afternoon will resolve the few problems that have emerged in recent months. Rob is convinced that the occasional slur in his speech is a side effect of the painkillers he is taking to help him cope with an old shoulder injury. He tells me he will be prescribed some new medication and that he'll be as right as rain within a week.

It's not raining, for once, on a mild December day in Leeds. Rob is waiting for me, full of smiles and good cheer as always, and I feel his strength and fitness surging through him as we hug. How could anything be wrong when he looks so well, and his body is still as lean and muscled as it was at the end of his rugby career?

Rob sounds happy after another enjoyable morning with the young Rhinos he is helping so much. It seems as if, after some testing times in his transition as a coach at the Leeds Academy, he has found his place. When he makes me laugh, I think how surreal it is that we are on our way to a medical consultation. As soon as we receive the all-clear, ordinary life can resume.

Our happiness had been dented during the October half-term break when we had taken the kids and my parents to our holiday home in Davenport, Florida. It was then that I first noticed how fatigued Rob had become.

We bought the villa – a twenty-minute drive from Disney World – soon after his testimonial season. Rob loves Disney, so much so that he proposed to me at a restaurant in Disneyland, Paris. I was so embarrassed that I spoilt it by ordering him to get up off his knee and sit down again. Rob was mortified and it took him another day to summon the courage to ask me in the more private setting of our hotel room. I loved that more discreet proposal and said an immediate 'yes'.

Even being told off by me did not curb Rob's Disney fairy tale and in 2012 he convinced me that the Davenport villa would be the ideal spot for future family holidays. We have since spoken about the possibility that, when we become old and grey together, we might even retire to the villa.

But all his usual zest for life was missing when we were in Davenport a few months ago. Rob was exhausted and I could tell how much it took for him to get out of bed and play with the kids. Sometimes I tried to persuade him to rest but Rob insisted he would be fine. He was able to summon some fresh energy and I decided that he was just worn out after the stress of his new job and preparing to move house.

His mum, Irene, and his former teammates had noticed a slight slur in his speech. Earlier that summer, when we were with his parents in Scotland, Irene had picked up on the way he stumbled over certain words. But she didn't say anything to me – and nor did Rob after an awards dinner for the Rhinos. He had gone up on stage that night in September and, before handing out a prize to one of the rising young stars from the Academy, had struggled to say 'consistency'. Kev Sinfield and others at the club were worried because they know that Rob is no drinker, so it was not a case of him having had a few too many beers. Understandably, they chose not to tell me.

I became aware of the problem when I heard how hard it was for Rob to say the word 'solicitor'. We were close to exchanging contracts on the sale of our house on Banbury Road and the purchase of our new home, not too far away in Pontefract. Rob was actually speaking to our solicitor when he kept tripping over that suddenly tricky word. It was then that I persuaded Rob to talk to the club doctor.

He already had an appointment to see the doctor because he was having considerable shoulder pain. Rob had broken his collarbone (or clavicle, to us physios), and had had a surgical procedure called an ORIF, or open reduction internal fixation. Screws and bolts kept the clavicle fixed in place, but, years later, the surgeons decided to remove the metalwork as his pain had intensified. As he was booked in to see the doctor for an injection, he agreed to also mention his speech problems.

I was worried when the doctor referred him to Nuffield Hospital in Leeds for an appointment with Dr Jeremy Cosgrove, a neurologist. The links between rugby and head trauma are well established and I understood why the club wanted to check for any early signs of dementia. The thought of Rob suffering from that slow yet terrible condition was distressing and, because the club had moved quickly in arranging a private consultation with an eminent neurologist, I went with him to Nuffield that Saturday morning.

The tests were thorough: after his bloodwork had been done, Rob underwent an MRI scan. The results would only be known in a week, but he also had numerous nerve conduction tests. I felt unsettled when, while sitting in on the consultation, it seemed to me that Rob's reflexes were a bit too brisk. A brisk reflex is never a good sign as it can indicate an upper motor neurone lesion. I tried to stay rational as it was just as likely that Rob was extremely anxious during the tests and was reacting with unnatural speed.

But, as a physio, I had treated patients with motor neurone disease before, so I asked Dr Cosgrove if it was possible that Rob had MND. He looked surprised and asked what gave me that idea. Had I been googling too much? I didn't bombard him with details of my professional experience with MND but listened instead as he reassured us that this was a very unlikely outcome. Motor neurone disease, he said, is a rare condition and he also thought Rob's age and fitness protected him. Dr Cosgrove suggested that Rob might be suffering from myasthenia gravis, which commonly affects the speech muscles, but he stressed that it was a treatable condition.

We felt relieved and Rob only began to worry when we heard nothing for more than a week. I decided to call the doctor's office and Dr Cosgrove's secretary quickly gave me good news: the MRI and bloodwork had all come back clear. They were just waiting for definitive results from the nerve conduction tests.

It had seemed to Rob and me that the MRI scan was the crucial examination. Once that came back free of any markers of neurological damage or trauma, relief flooded through us. Rob was so confident that everything would be okay, after he was prescribed the right medication, that he tried to persuade me that there was no need to disrupt my time with the kids. He suggested that he would see Dr Cosgrove in Leeds on his own while I picked up the girls from school and, early that evening, took them to their Thursday-evening swimming lessons.

It's obviously too important for me not to join Rob and, as my mum and dad are seeing a show in Manchester, my Auntie Sue has happily agreed to take care of the children this afternoon. So, rather than being filled with apprehension, I'm able to treat the idea of seeing the consultant as a positive. Once we get the appointment out of the way there will be an opportunity to spend a little time with Rob. Instead of changing Jackson's nappies or being a taxi driver for the girls, I will get to spend two or three hours with my husband.

Rob keeps up the wisecracks as we arrive at the hospital. We walk past Dr Cosgrove and, while he acknowledges us briefly, he avoids talking. I don't think too much about it and just assume he is busy and needs to start his appointments. In the waiting room, Rob keeps making me smile and I still feel hugely optimistic that everything will be resolved soon.

Our assumption comes to a shuddering halt a few minutes later. The doctor has been joined by a nurse and they look very sombre when we walk into his office. I feel sudden trepidation as I see their expressions. After he has introduced us to the nurse and listened to Rob's cheerful reply as to how well he is feeling, Dr Cosgrove speaks gravely.

He says how sorry he is to tell us that the news is not good. The doctor looks steadily at Rob, maintaining eye contact now, and says the fateful words. He thinks Rob has motor neurone disease because of the abnormal findings from the nerve conduction studies.

Rob looks at him blankly, because he has no idea of the severity of this sentence. It's very different for me. As soon as I hear the words 'motor neurone disease', it's as if a bomb has fallen from the sky and blown me wide apart. The bomb detonates deep inside me but, rather than erupting in an explosion of fire and noise, it spreads a far more terrifying silence. I know instantly that our glorious life together is over.

I find it difficult to look at Rob, the man I love and adore, because I understand far too clearly what it means. Rob will be buried alive in his own body. He will be trapped and paralysed beneath the rubble of MND.

The devastation will be so complete that, soon, he'll no longer be able to dress or feed himself or go to the toilet on his own. Even while his brain remains alert, and capable of deep cognitive thinking, a time will come when he can no longer talk or move. He will eventually struggle to breathe and be unable to swallow. An oxygen mask and an intravenous feeding tube will be the only ways to keep him alive – if such an existence can be called a life.

In a daze I listen as the doctor explains to Rob that MND is a progressive neurological condition that affects the brain and spinal cord. Messages from the brain to the rest of the body basically stop working, resulting in muscle weakness and then, ultimately, paralysis. Breathing and swallowing difficulties develop and, as the neurologist says with catastrophic finality, there is no cure.

He does not underline the fact that it is probably the cruellest disease of all but speaks instead about MND being such a complex affliction at cellular level. It is hard to comprehend why it affects only a small percentage of the population. I have since learned that an average of six people a day are diagnosed with MND in the UK – but the comparative rarity of the disease can be attributed to the fact that life expectancy is so drastically reduced.

For me it's the worst possible news. I am so distressed that I say silently to myself: *Please, no. Please, not this.*

I remember how many medical professionals have told me that MND is the one condition you need to avoid at all costs. Motor neurone disease locks you inside a body that doesn't function. I have seen such devastation with my own eyes on various hospital respiratory wards.

MND is a living death.

Rob, my husband and the sweetest, most loving man I have ever known, is about to enter the world of the living dead. I know there is no point in asking what can be done, because to do so will leave me furious with the initially evasive but ultimately futile answer: nothing. So I dredge up the residue of my shattered courage and ask about Rob's life expectancy.

Dr Cosgrove responds cautiously, because it is hard to make an exact prediction. But he then draws in a small breath and continues. Considering the test results, and the average statistics of similar cases, his honest prognosis is that Rob has eighteen months to two years of life left.

'I am so sorry,' he says quietly, before asking if we would like to talk in more detail with the nurse as we address our terminal future.

Rob is silent and so I shake my head. 'I just want to go,' I say bleakly.

We talk some more but I hear little of our desperate exchange. I am too busy clutching Rob's hand as I try to withstand the aftershocks of the bomb that has all but obliterated us. But, in my shell-shocked mind, the same questions rise up again and again.

How are we going to tell the children? What are we going to tell the children?

*

It's still light outside as we walk to the car, which Rob parked an hour earlier, when life still seemed full of hope and endless possibility. Everything has since changed. Rob puts his arm around me and, in his typical way, says: 'Thank God it's me – and not you or the children.'

This will always stay with me because Rob doesn't say: 'Why me?'

There is no self-pity and, as I am far more traumatised, he tries to lift me up. Rob looks at me soon after we get in the car. He has yet to turn on the ignition and he stretches out his hand to hold mine. 'It will be okay, Lindsey,' he says. 'We'll get through this.'

I squeeze his hand. I even try to smile but, on the inside, I think: *No, it's not going to be okay.*

I know what's coming and it feels as if my heart is about to crack into a thousand little pieces, bleeding shards of tissue and muscle, of broken love and shattered lives. Looking at Rob worrying about me, I nod. On the surface he is still glowing with health, but I have a sudden premonition of my incredible husband withered inside an immobile body.

I feel frightened for Rob. I see myself spooning mashed-up food into his mouth and struggling to wash him in the shower. I imagine lifting him up in my arms as I carry the dead weight of his body to bed. I hear myself chatting away to Rob even though, eventually, he will be as mute as I am now.

Tears roll down my cheeks and I allow myself to cry a little more as Rob holds me. When I eventually compose myself I see that his eyes are also glistening. But he's strong and he does not cry openly.

As we look helplessly at each other I feel a new surge of love. My heart is not broken after all. It's still pumping, for Rob, and I know that I am ready to care for him, tenderly and constantly, for however long we have left.

I lean over and kiss him, softly, on the cheek. Rob kisses me back.

The closeness between us helps, but then we bump into the ruins suddenly strewn around us. We talk of the kids and our parents. We will spare the children for as long as possible, but Rob is so worried about how his mum, and especially his dad, Geoff, might react to the news.

Rob means the world to his parents. Geoff, in particular, feels such pride in the way his tiny son shrugged aside the doubters who always dogged him. From his earliest junior years right the way through to all those Grand Finals, Rob ripped up presumptions that he was too small to ever make it. Instead, he has left a huge mark on rugby league and become one of the most cherished players in the country. Geoff has lived through each and every stage of Rob's struggles and triumphs. We know how crushed he will be to hear that we now face MND.

Geoff has recently had heart problems and Rob says: 'This could kill my dad.'

I drag myself out of the fog and point out that his parents had asked Claire and Joanne, Rob's sisters, to be with them as they waited for news. They will support Geoff and Irene.

'Your dad will be okay,' I say, trying to sound confident.

'You're right,' Rob says. 'I've got to tell them now.'

I can see how hard it is for Rob because he knows that a simple phone call will change his parents' lives for ever. Nothing can ever be the same again for them either.

Rob waits until we are out of the city and on the motorway. And then, when it's safe to make a hands-free call while driving, Rob hits the little green button to call his parents. I stare out of the window as we pass the darkening countryside. I love Yorkshire, and it's very beautiful, but it seems flat and featureless in the late-afternoon gloom.

On speakerphone we hear the phone ringing in Rob's family home. His parents have just a few seconds of peace left before the bombshell destroys them too.

Geoff answers and I am moved as I hear how carefully Rob speaks to his dad. He is extraordinarily calm as he explains the bad news. But the shock in Geoff's voice fills our car. We hear him talking to Irene and she starts crying. Geoff is so distraught that it sounds as if he has collapsed.

Claire comes on the line and Rob takes charge. He tries to reassure his sister and his parents. Rob tells them everything is going to be okay and that we will see them in another forty minutes. He also makes sure that his dad is all right.

I am just numb with grief.

But after Rob hangs up, I tell him how well he has done and that we will feel better once we are home. We then focus on the children and agree that we will not say anything to them until a few days after Jackson's birthday party on Saturday.

Rob says that we'll press ahead and make it the best possible party for Jackson, and the girls. We will also try to act as normally as possible. He's right and so I insist that I will take the girls to swimming this evening – which will give Rob more time with his parents.

I want to speak to my mum and dad but they have only just left Manchester – where they've been to the theatre to see *The Bodyguard*. It will be horrible for them to hear the news on a crowded train, so I decide to spare them a little longer.

The rest of the journey passes in a blur until we turn in to the drive of the Burrow family home. We have just got out of the car when Rob's parents and sisters come running out of the house. They hug us and, through a veil of tears and pain, Claire tells us not to worry. They will look after us and the children.

I am used to Claire and her big sister, Joanne, teasing Rob mercilessly. They have done this all his life because he is their little brother. It doesn't matter that they are proud beyond words that he became a rugby league superstar. They usually joke and kid around with Rob, and he is just as chirpy and cheeky in return. But this all stops now. Love and compassion pour from them, and from Geoff and Irene, and they can't stop crying and holding us.

Soon, it is time for me to drive across to my Auntie Sue. Slipping into practicality mode soothes me. Rob and I discuss logistics and agree that I will return to his parents with the children in a couple of hours and then we'll go straight home. But first, having hugged everyone again, I sit alone in the car and try to gather myself. It's important that I don't upset the children so I decide not to say a word to my aunt. I'll pretend that everything is fine.

It's easier than I expect because as soon as I arrive I am swept away by the chatter of the girls. They have so much to tell me about their day at school and how funny Jackson was when they were having their tea with Auntie Sue. I smile and laugh and cuddle them all, holding Jackson close while Sue helps Macy and Maya make sure they have everything.

Sue will look after Jackson a little longer while the girls are at swimming. It is all a whirl but the girls make it easier. They keep talking to me and each other as we drive through the dark. I don't think they notice how quiet I am compared to normal because they are still overflowing with news of their day.

I would break down if they were a little older and asked about their dad.

We make it to Featherstone, where their swim academy is held. It's black and freezing outside and the girls squeal as we run across to the light and warmth of the school. Once they are changed, and looking so lovely in their swimming costumes, I take them across to their respective classes. They barely give me a second glance as they are back with their friends.

I find a quiet place where, at last, I can call my mum. It's a few minutes after 6pm and she and Dad have just left Castleford station and are walking home. Mum immediately asks how we got on with the consultant.

She is so stunned when I tell her the news that she exclaims: 'You're joking!'

I'm not angry but I am pretty blunt, telling her that I wouldn't be ringing to make a joke about something so serious. I know she is plunged into a state of shock when she hears that Rob has been given less than two years to live.

She is quiet for so long that I have to say: 'Mum, are you still there?'

'I'm here,' Mum eventually says. She asks if she and Dad can come and see us tonight. I know how much I will need them in the months and years ahead and so I say it would be best if they wait until the morning. Rob and I will need some time alone once we get the kids to bed.

I only heard years later how devastated my parents had been. Too frightened to google MND, they sat up and talked and cried, and didn't sleep all night. My brother, Mark, came over to be with them for a few hours and he also couldn't believe it.

How could something so terrible happen to a person as good as Rob? What would happen to me and the children? Why did our family have to be torn apart?

My parents said later that they were 'dumbstruck', because they couldn't talk after a while. They sat in silence, mourning the loss of Rob, before they finally went to bed just before 4am. It didn't help. Their eyes remained wide open or filled with tears, until they could stand it no longer and got up again at six o'clock.

After I speak to Mum on the phone, I sit in a far corner of the spectator area overlooking the school swimming pool. I can't bear the thought of engaging in aimless chat with the other parents. So I keep my head down and start texting Rob.

I feel like a zombie, trying to process everything and stop myself from crying again.

The next two hours drift away in a shadowy haze. After swimming we pick up Jackson and then Rob. The five of us are finally home around 8pm.

Rob helps me put the children to bed and I am moved all over again as he says goodnight to each of them with almost unbearable tenderness. I know what he is thinking as we switch their lights off and slowly walk away.

Hours later, as we lie together in bed, quiet and unmoving despite being wide awake most of the night, these same questions roll through our heads. I stare into the darkness, wondering how much longer Rob will be able to bend down and kiss the children, let alone hold them. How much longer will he be able to say 'I love you' to Macy, Maya and Jackson? And how much time do we have left before he can no longer reach out to pull me close to him. How much time do we have left to talk and kiss and comfort each other? How many more nights will Rob, the love of my life, be with us?

2

The Birthday Party

I am proud to come from a Yorkshire coal-mining family. My dad, Graham Newton, and both my grandfathers, Alan Newton and Jimmy Bray, were all miners. They knew, with terrible intimacy, what it felt like to take the steel cage underground where they faced danger and fear. Conditions were cramped and difficult but they forged deep bonds with their fellow miners in the dusty dark. Once their long shifts were over, they would scrub themselves clean of the black streaks of coal and sink a few pints together at the local Miners' Welfare Club.

My dad was one of the 142,000 miners who went on strike against Margaret Thatcher and the National Coal Board in 1984 as they tried to stop the pit closures that eventually ripped apart towns such as Castleford, where I had been born two years earlier. I was obviously too young to understand how devastating those years were for my parents, and our entire community, but they were so destitute during the strike that they relied on soup kitchens and food hampers for many of our meals.

Both my grandads suffered underground. My dad's father,

Alan, had most of a finger amputated after a mining accident. In later life, he used his little stump to tease and playfully torment us as he prodded me and my brother, Mark, in the ribs. We would scream with delight when he wagged his deformed finger and chased us around the sitting room or the tiny garden. He was a great character. We called him Grandad Bully, and we loved him.

Grandad Jimmy, my mum's dad, had a scar on his back. It looked like the imprint of a giant shell, and it was far too pretty to really illustrate the horror of his ordeal underground. It was only years later that I grasped the enormity of all he endured. Until then he was just my lovely old grandad who would do anything for an easy life – even when under strict orders at home.

I always used to laugh because as soon as anyone walked through the front door, my Nana Nancy would say: 'Jimmy, put the kettle on . . . Jimmy, do this, Jimmy, do that.' He would jump up and do as he was told because he was just such a lovely, kind, caring and easy-going man. I thought the world of him, but Nana was definitely the boss.

My mum, Sharon, was the same. When she was still working in a nursery, where she was amazing with the little kids, she would leave my dad notes that said: 'Graham, here are your jobs for the day: tidy up the garden, go to the shops, cook the tea.' She was definitely in charge and kept my dad very busy in his early retirement.

It's in our family genes. The mum is always the boss and our poor old dads and husbands know it's best if they listen to us. We smile about it because it was the way in our house too. Rob, like Grandad Jimmy, is so relaxed – yet caring. I am the organised one, the practical partner who makes sure that everything gets done and that plans for the days, weeks and months ahead are in place.

As soon as I became Rob's full-time carer, as well as his wife, everything changed. The stories of Rob and Grandad Jimmy carried tragic similarities.

In 1969, Jimmy was involved in a terrifying accident at the Wheldale Colliery in Castleford. He and three other miners were working in the pit when a shaft collapsed. His close friend was struck on the head by a girder and fell down dead on top of Jimmy. A large portion of the pit then caved in on them, burying the men underground.

Jimmy was protected from most of the falling rubble by the body of the friend he had just lost. But he was still buried beneath a deep mound of the pit. It was frightening and suffocating because Jimmy and the two other survivors were trapped inside a black tomb of coal. The feeling of paralysis was especially acute for Jimmy because he was pinned down by a corpse.

Emergency excavation work began soon after the accident. But the men were buried so deep that hopes of a rescue faded with each passing hour. Twelve hours slipped away and, with still no sign of the men inside a graveyard of coal, the catastrophe was reported by the BBC and numerous national newspapers.

For Nana Nancy, my mum (who was only twelve years old) and her sister, Sue, Thursday afternoon and night were full of torment. They went down to the colliery to wait for news; after many futile hours they were advised to go home as hopes faded for the men. It was assumed that all four miners had perished beneath the avalanche of coal.

Reporters gathered outside their house that evening, hoping for some colour stories from a mining tragedy. My nana shut the door firmly as they waited and prayed.

The rescue teams kept digging and late that night a miracle happened: they uncovered Jimmy and the others. My mum and all the family cried with relief.

When they were finally reunited with Jimmy there was such elation because, as Mum later said, 'Your dad is your life, isn't he? We adored him and he adored us. And we had him back. He was alive and with us again.'

Jimmy had been through such incredible trauma and he only found the resolve to go on because, while buried alive, he visualised the future in his dazed mind. He imagined the weddings of his daughters, Sue and Sharon, and played them out, scene by scene. The pictures he dreamed up in his head, while struggling for breath, helped keep him alive, and he swore that, if he ever made it out of the pit, he would savour every hour of every day he had left as if it were his last.

Jimmy was scarred by the distressing incident – and not just physically. The shell I described on his skin had actually been a huge hole in his back caused by the crashing girders. But he waved away the concerns of his wife and children; he knew that the stitched-up wound would eventually heal. 'It's all right,' Jimmy would say. 'There's no need to fuss.'

Sharon and Sue could not stop staring at the hole in his back. Jimmy was quieter than normal but seemed to be recovering – only for the full extent of the psychological damage to emerge when he slept. My grandad had chilling nightmares and would wake screaming in the dead of night. For a while a lamp kept on on the bedside table helped, but the blood-curdling nightmares soon returned.

Nana Nancy was incredibly strong. The third of fourteen children, she had overcome hardship and poverty to build her own family. She helped Jimmy get better and kept everyone together.

Sharon and Sue were strong too. Whenever my nana asked them in the morning if they had managed to sleep, they said: 'Yes, Mam.' They would not reveal that they had been kept awake by the sounds of their father screaming and then crying in their mother's arms.

Grandad Jimmy never went down the mine again. He suffered from what we now call post-traumatic stress disorder and could only walk with callipers on his legs. But the colliery was good to him, and looked after our family, because Jimmy became the pit gardener. This seemed especially touching to me because there was no garden to be found anywhere among the slag heaps and dirt roads of the mine.

Only one of the three survivors took the cage down into the mine shaft again. But the stress caused him to suffer a massive heart attack and he was forced to retire on sick pay. The third miner became an invisible gardener alongside Jimmy.

My mum said that, from that moment on, she and Auntie Sue were brought up knowing life was precious. They were taught never to take it for granted and those lessons were passed on to me and Mark.

Of course, we were young and often forgot the value of life and good health, moaning about trivial things that held no lasting meaning. Rob and I split up when we were seventeen and for a couple of years we didn't see each other. That was my fault because I was silly when we had a teenage spat. I regretted it as soon as I took my haughty stance. But Rob came back into my life, when I least expected it, and put us back together again. For the next twenty-two years we were inseparable.

Now, having had Rob shackled by MND, I treasure life even more. I am given strength and hope by the remarkable positivity that Rob always showed even when he was buried inside his body, more harrowingly than Grandad Jimmy had been when trapped beneath his dead friend and a vast mountain of coal.

It seems almost profound that, exactly fifty years earlier, Grandad Jimmy's eerie foreshadowing of Rob's fate should have occurred. Just like my brave old grandad, my beautiful Rob clung to the remnants of life by making the most of the present and imagining a future full of love. I know that Rob, in another secret nod to Jimmy, was kept going by visualising the weddings of Macy, Maya and Jackson. Even though he would not be with us then, the sheer force of his will allowed Rob to endure three years beyond the initial prognosis. He witnessed so many milestones and achievements for the kids.

Through his determination and spirit, Rob also won awards and was honoured by the Royal Family, the government and the country at large.

His courage and resilience came from deep within his stricken body and, even more than wonderful old Grandad Jimmy, he inspired and lifted me every day.

But, at the beginning of this brutal struggle against MND, we were hopelessly raw and vulnerable. We soon learned simple yet immense lessons of life. Rather than feeling sorry for ourselves, as we did at the start, we understood that there could still be joy amid the grief, and enough light and laughter to sweep away the darkness and the tears we buried deep inside ourselves.

We just needed time to reach such acceptance.

Friday 13 December 2019, Pontefract

My mum and dad arrive around ten o'clock. It is the morning after the diagnosis. Sleepless and emotional, Mum's eyes are glazed when Rob opens the door. She and Dad walk sadly into our new home. She hugs me and so does my dad.

After Rob accepts her embrace he speaks firmly to Mum. 'No tears, Sharon,' he says. 'We're not crying because it's not going to help any of us. We'll cope with this. We'll survive. We've all got each other and we will be fine.'

Mum and Dad both murmur: 'We will . . . we will.'

They don't know how we will ever be fine again but they

want to help in any way they can. Mum asks about Macy and Maya and Rob says he took them to school this morning, as normal. We will carry on and help the kids feel as if nothing has changed and that everyone is safe and well, especially with Jackson's party tomorrow.

Rob sounds so strong but then, in this moment of forced composure, Jackson toddles into the living room. He has only been walking for a few weeks and he is very unsteady on his chubby little legs. Rob instinctively scoops him up in his arms. The close contact with our beautiful boy cracks Rob open.

Holding Jackson, Rob breaks his own rule. Tears stream down his face as he looks at me and my parents. 'I'm never going to see him grow up, am I?' he says.

We have no answer. We just stand there, dumb witnesses to Rob's terrible pain.

'I'll be okay,' Rob says as I try to comfort him. 'Just give me a moment.'

He walks across to the far window. Jackson babbles happily in his dad's arms as Rob gazes at our back garden where he recently put up a trampoline and slide for the kids.

I lead Mum and Dad into the kitchen, to give Rob some privacy. Dad normally doesn't show too much emotion but now he looks like an open wound. He and Mum are sluffened – an old word that slips into my head. It means they are devastated or sickened with sadness.

'I wish it was me,' Dad says. 'I wish it was me and not Rob.'

Mum tries to echo Rob as she says we are going to be all right. I speak up, with a sharp edge to my voice, sounding so unlike myself – usually, I talk calmly and cheerfully. But all my calm and cheer have been blown to smithereens.

'I know what this disease is, Mum,' I say angrily. 'I know what's going to happen to Rob.'

I shake my head, in desolation, and repeat those words. 'I know what's going to happen.'

But I can no longer support myself. I collapse and, unable to keep Rob's rule either, cry hysterically. I can't stop for a long time and my mum and dad, their knees pressed against the cold hard kitchen floor, just hold me.

After a while they help me to my feet. Mum gives me a handful of tissues to wipe my eyes and Dad puts the kettle on. I lean against the work surface so that I don't fall down again.

Mum and Dad are numb, and as heartbroken as me. I can see what I've done to them and it feels bad. It helps no one, least of all Rob, being sluffened.

Since that horrible Friday morning, neither Rob nor I have broken down in front of anyone else. We tried to find hope and happiness, even in the smallest and most unexpected of places, even though MND is such a grim and relentless disease.

As I return to the front room, after my tears in the kitchen, I smile at Rob and Jackson. Rob smiles back and walks over to me.

'I love you,' he says quietly as he wraps an arm around me.

'I love you too,' I reply, in a voice filled with conviction rather than crying and snuffling.

I kiss Rob, and then Jackson too. Rob squeezes me tightly, and reassuringly.

'Tomorrow,' he promises, 'we'll give this little man a party to remember ... '

My best friend, Angela Elsworth, lived with her husband, Ross, and their son, Alexander, in Bedale, a lovely little market town in the Yorkshire Dales. Bedale is fifty miles north of Pontefract and, despite being seven months pregnant with her second child, William, Angela said she was never going to miss Jackson's first birthday party. We had been pregnant with our boys at the same time, and Alexander was just two months older than Jackson, but our friendship ran far deeper than just that connection.

Rob and I had known Angela for over twenty years and we had been on countless holidays together. It seemed strange to think that Rob first met Angela without me. I was at university in Manchester, after my fleeting break-up with Rob, and one of his close friends at the time, Steven Varley, was going out with Angela.

When she met Rob, Angela couldn't believe his boundless energy or how small he was for a rugby player. She was eighteen, and Rob was nineteen going on nine. As they sat and watched in Steven's front room, Rob kept doing forward rolls on the carpet. He was just so full of life and tricks. Rob soon had Angela out on the local school field playing rugby with him and Steven. She loved it and so when Rob and I got back together in my second year at uni, we struck up a great friendship.

Some of our best holidays before we got married were with Angela. That continued after she met Ross, and we still talk fondly of breaks we had as couples together in the Dominican Republic and Thailand. Angela still cracks me up to this day when she recounts some of Rob's high points and mishaps on our vacations over the years.

Once, in the Dominican Republic, Rob was reluctant to join in a party game the hotel had organised to see who could throw a watermelon the furthest into a huge swimming pool. All these big men were flexing their muscles and giving it everything as they hurled the watermelon. Finally, when it was Rob's turn, he shocked everyone but us by flicking it way beyond the pool to win the prize. But he was more comfortable just being my Rob.

In Thailand he had us rocking with laughter after a stint of bartering for some shoes he fancied. He eventually came away with the shoes but grinned in embarrassment when he realised he had offered more than the initial asking price. On a different holiday Rob decided to pack all the beers left in the hotel mini-bar so he could take them as a gift to his grandad. This was way back when you could still bring liquids on to a plane, so he crammed all the beers into his carry-on luggage. The bag was so stuffed that it split open, and glass got smashed and cut the leg of a St Helens fan who just happened to be standing behind us in the passport queue. Fortunately, the Saints supporter laughed off the tiny cut caused by the smallest Rhino in the Leeds squad.

I was even scattier than Rob. We spent an afternoon one New Year's Eve with Angela and Ross in Bedale as we were on our way to a family party. When Rob asked me for the postcode, just as we were about to leave Angela's, his face was a picture when he found the address on his phone. I had told him that we were going to a family party in Durham and that we could stop off at Angela's as Bedale was on the way.

'I thought we were going to Durham?' Rob said reasonably.

'Yes,' I said brightly. 'We're going to Newark.'

'Lindsey,' Rob said with rare exasperation, 'we go past Newark on the train down to London. We've driven an hour in completely the wrong direction.'

'Geography has never been my strong point,' I admitted as everyone, even Rob, laughed.

Angela and I went on girly holidays together, with our mutual friend Vicky, and they would laugh so much because I always sang the wrong words to certain songs. I would go off for a run, with my trusty old iPod and headphones, and they would hear me coming back singing along to 'Peggy Sue' by Buddy Holly. The only problem was that I would be singing 'Begging you' instead of 'Peggy Sue.'

They'd whoop with amusement as, in a loud, breathless and probably off-key voice, I sang:

> *'Begging you, begging you*
> *Oh, how my heart yearns for you.'*

I wasn't remotely bothered when, as patiently as they could amid the laughter, Angela and Vicky told me that it really was a song about a girl called Peggy Sue. I now know that it was released in 1957, so I like to think that Grandad Jimmy and

Nana Nancy might have bopped away to it – while probably singing the right words.

One of the many reasons why I love Angela is that she is always amused by my kooky quirks. On my way to her hen party in 2017, I had a crazy journey. In an old text we smiled at recently, I told Angela:

> I am on the train, should get to Liverpool for 10am. I've had a very stressful start as I nearly missed my train. Didn't realise that all the city centre roads are closed due to the Tour de Yorkshire so got lost and couldn't find anywhere to park. I literally ran through Leeds (without my shoes on), lost a flip flop en route, fell running across the road and scuffed my jacket but on a positive I made my train and looking forward to spending the day with you all xx.

We loved going to gigs together – from Alicia Keys and Beyoncé to Kylie and Girls Aloud – having fancy afternoon teas and spa days. It tickled Angela when, in our early days together, I always made Rob return any designer gift he bought me from Harvey Nichols in Leeds. He once gave me a Gucci handbag and I refused to accept it, telling him: 'Rob, I'm not a Gucci girl. I'm happy with ASOS.'

Rob was actually relieved that I was not into anything outrageously expensive – even if he and Angela liked to remind me that I could be extravagant when it came to our house on Banbury Road. Angela and Ross had once lived right around the corner from us on Wiston Drive. We spent a fortune on the fireplace in our old house (I had to have a chimney installed so I could have the fire I so desperately wanted), and then I made a poor old tiler remove all the mosaic tiles I had asked him to use to cover one wall of our bathroom. As soon as I saw the finished work I decided they were all wrong and made him take them down and eventually start again with some replacement tiles.

Soon after we got that house perfect, Rob and I decided to put an offer in on our current home. And then MND came along and made all those crazy little indulgences redundant. We were locked in to a terminal illness rather than scouring ASOS or the online tile stores.

It was hard to think of anything else, even on the day our little boy had his first birthday party.

Saturday 14 December 2019, Pontefract

Angela's family are among the first guests to arrive and Rob welcomes them to the party. I am busy with Jackson and making last-minute preparations and so I don't see Angela for a while. I've resolved not to mention our news because even saying the words 'Rob has MND' out loud would turn me into a blubbering wreck again. It's vital that I focus on Jackson and the other children and make sure they have a special afternoon.

Rob takes a different approach. As he trusts Angela so much he tells her about the diagnosis. He does not share his death sentence and so Angela, who knows very little about MND, nods sympathetically without really understanding the nature of our personal disaster.

She says a heartfelt sorry without adding anything else. Her attention is also diverted by her son, Alexander, pointing to the coloured balloons, which say 'Happy Birthday Jackson'. Angela apologises to Rob and says she will find him later to have a proper chat.

Adult conversations rarely happen at children's parties and Angela doesn't talk properly to me or Rob this afternoon. It suits me just to engage in amiable chit-chat with everyone before I'm called away to sort something out with the cake, party bags or my own two girls, looking so grown up compared to the large group of gurgling babies and toddlers who are overwhelmed by the experience.

But the new gravity of our lives is rarely far away. I see Rob sitting with Jackson on his lap, his face creased with jumbled emotions. Later, I glance across at his dad, Geoff, gazing into the distance, his eyes swimming with tears.

When the time comes to sing, 'Happy Birthday', Rob and I smile, with Jackson propped on my hip, and our two voices rise up above everyone else's. Angela begins to worry as she notices that half the adults at the party are singing with gusto, while the other half, including the grandparents, are struggling to hold back the tears.

She speaks briefly to my mum who confirms that the news is not good, without giving away many more details. It's only late this afternoon, following all the thanks and goodbyes, that Angela can talk to her husband as they drive back to Bedale with Alexander fast asleep in his car seat.

When Ross hears the letters MND he looks over at his wife in shock. 'Angela, that's really serious,' he says.

Ross's expression has changed so much that Angela feels a shiver run through her. 'What is it?' she asks.

Ross finds a safe spot to pull over. He glides to a stop and switches off the engine.

Alexander is still asleep. Ross opens his phone and taps 'MND' into the search engine.

He explains the basic facts and then hands his wife the phone after a few minutes. The car is quiet as Angela reads.

'Oh my God,' she finally says, the shock and horror making her voice ragged. She begins to cry and the tears soon turn to sobs.

Ross leans across to Angela and holds her. He has no words to say right now apart from, 'I'm sorry, Ange . . . I am so, so sorry.'

The kids are winding down after all the excitement, watching a cartoon on television, while I reach for my phone. Rob has just told me that he spoke to Angela. I feel relieved. It's best my friend knows the truth. Rob also mentions that Angela didn't seem to quite understand the magnitude of our news. He knows why because, just a few days ago, Rob himself did not fathom the catastrophic meaning of MND.

I type words on my screen, trying to help explain everything while remaining calm. It takes a few minutes and then I send this message:

Hi Angela, thank you for coming today. It was lovely to see you. I'm sorry I couldn't tell you face to face today cos we wanted it to be a good/happy day for Jackson. We got some devastating news on Thursday. Rob has been having some problems with his speech and muscle twitches. He's been having some tests and they've diagnosed him with motor neurone disease. It's not good news. They said he may have 1–2 years. It's a life-limiting disease and there is no cure. I'm absolutely heartbroken and I can't talk about it just yet – it's too raw. But I just wanted to let you know. I'm sorry I forgot your presents they are all wrapped and ready to give you but my mind is all over the place xxx

At 17:29 my phone pings. It's Angela:

It was such a lovely party hun. Jackson is such an amazing little boy, you are all being incredibly strong.

Rob mentioned it to me when we were talking at the party but I will be honest I didn't know what motor neurone disease was and didn't want to ask too much as I could tell it was hard to talk about. Ross googled it in the car and we are both absolutely heartbroken for you. We had to pull over because I was shaking so much. I feel awful now for how I reacted when Rob mentioned it, but I just had no idea it was so terrible.

We love you both so very much and although we don't see each other as often as we should, I regard you as one of my closest friends.

We are both completely devastated for you and so stunned. I have no idea how you all got through today. We feel so helpless but I mean it from the bottom of my heart when I say we are here if you need anything at all. Please just ask.

Please do not even apologise about forgetting presents that is really not important.

Sending you all of our love and prayers xxxx

At 17:57 I send my reply:

I'm so sorry I couldn't tell you in person, I wanted to, I really did but I knew if I said anything I would break down and we said today was about Jackson and we wanted to make some happy memories for him. It just doesn't seem real. I'm just so sad that Rob won't be here to see the kids grow up and it's breaking my heart.

Thank you for your message it means a lot. You are a special friend. Look after those beautiful boys of yours xxx

♥

At 18:10 there is one more WhatsApp message from Angela:

You don't have to apologise for not telling me in person at all. I have absolutely no idea how you are keeping it together. You both did Jackson so proud, he had a fabulous time.

I know what you mean about it not feeling real. He is just so young. It's unbelievably unfair. I cry every time I think about how much he is going to miss. Life can be so cruel.

Please let me know if I can do anything, we don't have to talk about anything you don't want to, but I have so many hugs waiting for you xxx

I read the words, swallow my tears and shut my phone down. I look across at Rob and smile. He smiles back.

'It was good, wasn't it?' I say.

Rob knows I am talking about the party. His smile turns into a grin. 'It was great,' he says before pointing at the three sleepy children spread out on the carpet in front of us. 'And they loved it. That's what matters.'

I walk across to hug and kiss my dying husband. We hold each other for a long time and then, nodding and smiling at Rob, I turn to the kids.

'Right, you three,' I say cheerfully. 'It's time for a bath, a story to read in bed and then sleep.'

'Can we have five more minutes?' eight-year-old Macy asks. 'It is Jackson's birthday.'

'Ten?' her four-year-old sister asks more hopefully.

'What do you think, Rob?' I say with a little laugh, 'Five more minutes?'

Rob pauses, stretching out the moment as the girls look at their dad expectantly. 'Ten more minutes sounds good to me,' he eventually suggests.

Maya and Macy start cheering. Rob's smile widens, lighting up his face from within, as he says, 'It's a special day, after all.'

3

Castleford Days

My mum and dad remember the queues but, most of all, they remember how they tried to make me feel excited and special. In the bleak winter of 1984, nine months into the year-long miners' strike, I was just two years old. But the old family story of how my parents reacted to the hardship and deprivation resonates all these decades later. Seeing the long, snaking lines of people in front of them, they would laugh and make it a surprise treat for me.

'Oh, look, Lindsey,' my mum would exclaim, 'the café's really busy today!'

'Yeah,' my dad would say with a chuckle. 'They must have something really tasty for our tea.'

They turned the bitter conflict with Margaret Thatcher and the National Coal Board, which left them destitute and worried, into a game. The 'café' was actually a soup kitchen at the Methodist church hall on Carlton Street in Castleford.

I have heard them recount their memories so often that I can almost see the images of the soup kitchen and the crowds of hungry families in my head forty years later. I can imagine myself as a little girl, enjoying those moments as if they were thrilling social occasions rather than desperate times.

Of course, I now understand how difficult the strike was for my parents and so many mining communities across the country. There had once been a thousand coal mines in Britain, but the number of working pits had shrunk to a mere 173 at the start of 1984. Thatcher wanted to go much further by shutting down the remaining mines while breaking the National Union of Mineworkers – all part of a campaign to shatter the wider labour movement. She was determined to achieve her aims no matter the cost to mining families. She did not seem to care that, away from the mines, there was little work for anyone in towns like Castleford.

Apart from the severe threat of redundancy, the miners and their wives recognised that their towns and villages would be on the brink of collapse if the surrounding collieries were closed. The slogan that was used so often by the strikers and their supporters carried a simple yet powerful message: 'Close a pit, kill a community.'

My dad had started working in the mines at sixteen, in 1974, when he earned a weekly wage of £17. His salary had increased to £120 a week by the time he and tens of thousands of other miners went on strike against the pit closures in March 1984. This was a modest wage for work so dangerous and exhausting that, even now, my dad describes it with great care.

Dad always says how lucky he was not to work at the coalface. He was a blacksmith welder at Allerton Bywater colliery, just a few miles from our home in Castleford, and so most of his work was done above ground. My dad wore a big black helmet and visor as he used the extreme heat of the forge to soften the iron and metal hooks and handles of the carriages and pulleys. He knew that when the fiery red heat turned to a prettier yellowy-orange the iron had become softer and more pliable. Dad then used his hammers and chisels to bend, reshape and fuse pieces of metal with an almost magical touch.

He prepared the conveyors and repaired the damaged chutes and cords, trolleys and little coal trains that became dented and broken during the constant shuttle of work. But a few times a week my dad had to go down into the pit to carry out repairs underground. He told me in later years how scared he felt stepping into the cage, which would then drop beneath the surface. Down they would sink, in a two-minute ride to the bottom, as fear lurched inside them with every bump and rattle of the cage.

The first time my dad went underground he was amazed to find that the pit was lit up. He had been expecting it to be completely dark and dingy. Instead, his initial thought was that he had discovered an underground hotel because it was so light and so busy. But, with the air dusty and the conditions cramped, this was no hotel.

Some coalfaces were so excruciatingly hot that shirtless miners worked in shorts as the coal-streaked sweat poured off them. At other places underground it was so wet and cold that the men pulled on more clothes to stop their overalls, and themselves, becoming drenched. And then, worst of all, there were the pitch-black shafts. The only light in the otherwise impenetrable darkness came from the small torches attached to their helmets. They shone like quivery pinpricks in the inky blackness.

Dad felt such relief that he didn't have to work there. Men crawled through the shafts, bumping against the wooden chocks that stopped the roof from caving in on them. Even if the miners had been less than three feet tall they would have still had to slither across the surface before they dug for coal on their hands and knees. Some of their shifts lasted for twelve hours.

Tragically, not everyone came back alive when the cage returned to the surface. Dad lost two friends underground, Malcolm King and Keith Carter. The welders worked on the tops of cages without harnesses, which my dad hated. He said being unattached to the cage was far worse than going down into the deepest part of the mine. They would teeter on the swaying cage, changing the wire ropes, and every step felt like a gamble with life. It was only after Keith was hit by a girder and knocked down the shaft to his death, that the bosses supplied harnesses to make the men feel safer.

My dad would grease the cage ropes and clean out the ring dams around the shaft, which were meant to stop water cascading down on the miners. It was messy work but Dad never complained. He and my mum accepted that mining had been part of our family history for generations and that it gave us food to eat and put a roof over our heads. It also bound our community tightly together.

When I was seven years old and my brother Mark was four,

my parents took us to a disused pit in Wakefield, which had
been turned into a kind of museum in honour of the abandoned mining industry. We sank down into the cold and the
dark in a cage and, while we clung to Mum, Dad grinned. I
didn't like it – it really was scary. When we reached the bottom,
it didn't look much like a hotel to me; it looked like a horrible
cave full of unimaginable terrors.

Mark was even more agitated. 'Mum,' he whispered urgently,
'I need a wee.'

After Mum told him that he would just have to hold on as
there were no toilets underground, Mark asked a perfectly
reasonable question: 'What did Grandad do if he wanted the
toilet?'

Everyone laughed, which made Mark squirm even more.
But I also thought of poor Grandad Jimmy and how he must
have felt while he was buried alive for so long underground. I
just wanted to get out of the black hole and feel the pale and
watery Yorkshire sun on my skin – while Mark and Mum
rushed to the loo.

Years before seeing that snapshot of working life for both
my grandfathers, and my dad, I was protected from the harsh
struggle my parents endured during the strike. Mark had not
been born then and Mum, Dad and I lived in a small two-
bedroom house on Lock Lane, half a mile from the Castleford
soup kitchen.

By digging in to their savings, they managed to pay the
monthly mortgage but not much money was left over for food
and bills. They had to rely on their parents for help and the

soup kitchen for sustenance. Once a month they queued up for food hampers donated to the miners by countries from around the world – including the old Soviet Union. The hampers offered very basic food but Mum and Dad always said they could make meals out of almost anything.

While they were anxious about money, and worrying about how the miners could keep resisting a merciless government, my parents made the most of life. Mum had given up work to look after me and she loved having Dad around to spend time with us rather than at the colliery. They went on long walks, pushing me in my buggy, and felt lucky to be alive and above ground. Dad also started to run and became really fit, eventually running his first London Marathon in 1986, when I was four. During the strike he would often happily disappear for a ten-mile run.

One of those runs gave us another famous Newton family story from the strike. Dad had run about six miles when, in the distance, he saw a man digging in a field. He kept running and soon passed a parked car, which looked suspiciously like the old banger owned by his father – or Grandad Bully as I called him. Dad fixed his gaze on the man digging and then came to a stop.

'Dad!' he cried out. 'What are you doing?'

Grandad Bully stopped digging and looked up. 'What do you think I'm doing?' he said as he gestured at the freshly dug potatoes strewn around his muddy boots.

'But they're not your potatoes,' my dad said.

'No,' Grandad Bully agreed thoughtfully, 'but we need to eat.'

My dad just laughed and decided to join his father in the field. Together, they stuffed two bags full of potatoes. When they drove back to Lock Lane, with the sweat drying on Dad's beaming face, they gave my mum such a shock.

'What am I going to do with all these potatoes?' she asked.

'I would eat them if I were you,' Grandad Bully said helpfully.

For the next few weeks we followed Grandad Bully's advice and ate our potatoes. Mum surprised us with the versatility of the humble potato. We ate mashed potato, chips, jacket potatoes, boiled potatoes, cottage pie, sautéed potatoes and even potato salad. This creativity, positivity and resilience defined my parents, and Castleford itself, and meant that I had a blissfully happy childhood, despite the strike and its aftermath.

When the dispute finally ended, amid great heartache in March 1985, my parents refused to be downtrodden. My dad went back to work and, when he picked up his first weekly wage from the pit in a year, he came back to celebrate with Mum and me.

Mum opened the little brown envelope which had 'Graham Newton' written on it. Inside there were fourteen £10 notes. £140 a week marked a small raise from a year before. Mum carefully put the money back into the envelope and then she waved it cheerfully above my head.

'Look, Lindsey,' she said as Dad laughed. 'We're millionaires!'

My mum always tells me that I was a very contented baby. It helped that she was confident, despite being a new mother, so when I was sleeping peacefully in those first few hours after my birth she resisted the urging of the nurses to wake me up. Mum insisted that I would start crying when I was hungry. And of course I did. It was the same when I got home. The community nurse would come check on my progress and, while I slept through her visit, she peered into the cot and saw how serene I looked.

That calm confidence shaped my childhood too. I was walking at nine months and by the time I went to nursery I was different to some of the other children. While many of them were crying as their mothers helped them take their coats off, I apparently walked ahead. I just took my coat off and hung it up. One of the nursery teachers said to my mum: 'She's so independent and confident . . . that's good.'

My mum smiled and replied: 'That's our Lindsey.'

We had moved by then to our current family home in Castleford, soon after Mark was born, and I often played with my friend Sally Price who lived in the house behind us. We liked playing in their garden; at the end of the afternoon Sally was always immaculate while Mrs Price often looked embarrassed as she handed me back over the fence. She was more prim and proper than Mum and so she would always apologise and say: 'I'm ever so sorry, Sharon. I don't know what happened to Lindsey.'

Mum just laughed because I would be covered in mud after such a fun afternoon.

My parents and I laugh together now when we see how Maya, my younger daughter, always gets so filthy when she is playing with paints or outside in the garden.

Macy and Maya are also like me as they love singing and dancing – with the distinct difference that they are really talented performers. I had none of their ability, but I made up for it with enthusiasm. I was a great fan of musicals and my mum took us to the theatre in London to see *Joseph and the Amazing Technicolour Dreamcoat*. We sat behind Shirley Bassey, who was there with her grandchildren, and we had photographs taken with her after the show.

I also remember my mum taking me to a Take That concert as I had their posters, including a special pin-up of Mark Owen, on my bedroom wall – alongside Ryan Giggs as well as Jason Donovan and Kyle Minogue (I loved *Neighbours*). I was also crazy about *Friends*, which was first shown in the UK in 1995 when I was twelve years old. But a coffee shop in Manhattan seemed very different to school in Castleford. Ryan Giggs, living closer to me in Manchester, seemed more familiar.

My dad was a Leeds United season ticket holder and he was happy to bore anyone with his memories of the great team Don Revie managed in the 1960s and '70s. But names like Billy Bremner, Norman Hunter and Jack Charlton meant nothing to me. Ryan Giggs was different and dreamy and when Dad asked if I wanted to go with him and Mark to a game between Leeds and Manchester United, I was ecstatic.

I spent a good hour getting ready. When I came downstairs, saying how excited I was to be seeing Ryan Giggs, my dad looked horrified. He ordered me to take the red ribbons out of my hair, which I had chosen just for Ryan and Man United, or I could stay at home. I was really put out and couldn't understand the fuss about silly old Leeds as they weren't much good anyway. But I did as I was told.

So I saw Ryan Giggs play but I wasn't allowed to say another word about him. Unsurprisingly, my dad never invited me to the football again.

I was more interested in dance classes anyway, as an eager if limited member of Noreen's Dance School in Castleford. Claire and Joanne Burrow were the best dancers there; when we did ballroom, I was always happy if Jo was my partner. Their little brother, Rob, was often there when they were picked up by their mum, Irene.

Rob was small but I thought he was cute. He seemed to always wear the blue-and-amber colours of the Leeds Rhinos. It was quite a statement because Castleford was a passionate rugby league town and our fans hated the Rhinos.

But I learned that Rob, like his dad, had loved the Rhinos all his life and, aged twelve, he had signed a contract to join the Leeds Academy. I wasn't that impressed as I had no idea then that Rob dreamed of becoming a professional rugby player. We never spoke to each other at first because we were both so shy and went to different schools. I was at Castleford High while Rob went to Airedale High, a mile and a half down the road.

I think Rob only really noticed me when we were about fourteen and he was dragged along to a presentation even-ing at Noreen's after we had done our dance exams. We were milling around afterwards, chattering away, and for some reason I asked: 'Does anyone know how Cas got on this afternoon?'

It was a strange question from me because I really didn't care too much if the Castleford Tigers won or lost – but I thought of them as my team because Mum and Dad had always supported them and the Cas ground at Wheldon Road, which everyone called The Jungle, was a four-minute drive from our house.

At that mention of rugby, Rob looked over with interest. I was the girl who danced with his big sister – one of two sisters who teased and tormented him constantly. So I suddenly registered with him and he decided I was pretty. I knew nothing about this at the time, but Rob came over to tell me all about the game and how Castleford had done. We were both more interested in each other than the score.

Not too long after that conversation, Rob asked me out to the movies. It felt like it was a date, so I said yes. But our plans were spoiled because of a mutual friend called Glenn; my mum was also friends with Glenn's mum and word soon got out. Glenn's mum told her that Rob and I were going to the movies together, and when Mum asked me about it I was mortified and flatly denied it. I don't know why I did because Mum wouldn't have minded. We knew the Burrows well, so Rob obviously came from a good family.

But once I had assured Mum that I was most definitely not going out on a date with Rob Burrow, there was no changing tack. I felt too bad to call Rob and tell him the truth and so, to my shame, I stood the poor boy up. I think he waited outside Carlton Lanes Shopping Centre in Castleford for a good half-hour, hoping that I'd finally show up so that we could travel together to the cinema in Wakefield. We didn't speak about it when I saw him the next time at Noreen's, but I really should have said 'I'm so sorry, Rob.'

There was another chance about a year later. Glenn was going out with my friend Kim and the boys had a chat about me. Glenn told Rob that I had mentioned to Kim that, maybe, I had made a mistake in missing our first date. Rob was keen to give it another try and so Kim suggested a double date to me. I said yes again, and this time I didn't back out.

The four of us caught a bus to Wakefield – there still wasn't a cinema in Castleford – and Rob was funny and kind. All my nerves disappeared. Rob wore a leather jacket, which I was convinced belonged to his dad. It was far too big for him and he looked like he was drowning inside it. In later years he assured me the jacket was actually his and I believed him because I knew by then that Rob loved *Grease*. He fancied himself as Castleford's answer to Danny Zuko, even if John Travolta was just a tad taller than Rob.

But the most touching moment of the date came when we left the cinema and Rob offered me his jacket to keep warm. I said no because I really didn't want to be seen walking around Wakefield in a leather jacket that looked as if it belonged to Rob's dad. But I appreciated the gesture because it showed that, even at fifteen, Rob was very thoughtful.

I also discovered that he was quite vulnerable when the four of us went for a pizza before we caught the bus back to Castleford. We started talking about names, for some reason, and Glenn made Rob blush. He turned to Rob and said: 'We'll avoid talking about middle names.' Of course that made Kim and I want to know more. It turned out that Rob's full name was Robert Geoffrey Burrow. His middle name came from his dad, Geoff, but Rob hated being called 'Geoffrey' so he tried to keep it a secret. I felt for him as he flushed red with embarrassment.

I changed the subject to help Rob, because I liked him, and from that point it just felt right. Rob became my boyfriend soon afterwards.

We were good together even though we were very different. Rob was full of high jinks and mischief with his friends, while I was much more studious – perhaps even boring compared to the cool kids. I loved school and I worked hard. I remember how, one year, we came home from a long-awaited holiday abroad the day that the school term at Park Juniors started. While Mark told Mum he was too exhausted to go in after we got back around lunchtime, I was out the door, in my uniform, and on the way to school within fifteen minutes of our return home.

I was not the brightest in my class, but my marks were good because I was so conscientious. Rob was much more of a free spirit who was obsessed with rugby. He was never a big talker, though, and he downplayed his ambitions to become a professional with the Rhinos.

In my own way I was also quietly driven. For a long time, as a young girl, I had wanted to become a PE teacher. But too many cold and rainy mornings in Castleford put me off the idea and soon a different path emerged in my head. Mark was a very good footballer and had joined the Barnsley Academy. Some weekends I was dragged along to watch; for me the tedium was lifted whenever I saw the physiotherapist at work with the boys. It immediately appealed because I like helping people, and I like science and medicine, and some sport too.

I began to consider it more seriously as our GCSEs loomed. My determination was sharpened when one of my teachers heard that I was thinking about going to university to study physiotherapy so I could eventually work in the NHS. He said that I needed to be really strong in the sciences and suggested that this would be a step too far for me. Even if I did well in my GCSEs, there was no chance I would get an A* and a couple of As at A-level.

That hurt but it also steeled me. I thought: *I'll show you . . .*

While I worked even harder at school it was different for Rob. His mum was really worried that Rob would not pass any of his GCSEs; before most of his exams, she would tear her hair out because he had forgotten his pen or pencil and ruler. Before his art exam he had had to borrow coloured pencils from his friends at school. They could only spare the rubbish colours, like brown, because they needed the more vibrant ones for their own work.

I didn't know whether to be amused or scandalised when Rob told me what he had done in his religious education exam. Asked to draw an artistic impression of God, Rob sketched a figure of a man in a Leeds Rhinos kit.

Rob did well enough in the end and, to his mum's relief, got seven GCSEs. He was very impressed by my twelve GCSEs but he didn't need as many because he was about to sign a professional contract with the Rhinos. It was more important for me as I looked ahead to my A-levels and a career in physiotherapy. I was a step closer to showing that harsh teacher I could get the grades I needed to go to a good university.

I began my A-levels at New College in Pontefract in late 1999. Life with Rob was fun for the whole of the next year until, suddenly and inexplicably, he let me down. We were nearly eighteen and Rob had spoilt me by buying me a champagne gold Nokia phone. They were those old bricks where you had to press a number on the phone numerous times to get the right letter when you were sending a text. 'Champagne gold', meanwhile, was simply the colour rather than a fancy phone. But I loved it; and Rob and I often sent messages when we were not together.

One day, however, we had an argument over a really trivial misunderstanding. I got needlessly angry and told Rob I was breaking up with him. It was over.

Rob looked really hurt but no amount of apologising from him could change my mind. That was it. We were finished.

I regretted it almost as soon as I said the words, but I couldn't easily back down. I had to live with my mistake. Then, after a few days of missing him like crazy, I messaged Rob to ask if we could talk. He didn't answer and so I took to calling his landline at home. I could hear how awkward his dad sounded when he said Rob was out. I think he was just trying to cover for Rob who, clearly, was avoiding me. When I phoned again a few days later, Claire answered. She was friendly and said to hang on while she called Rob to the phone.

But even that didn't work. Rob told Claire that he didn't want to talk to me.

I felt devastated. It was all my fault for being so cold and angry when Rob made a silly mistake that no longer mattered.

Rob had chosen to show me the truth of my words. It really was over.

My family loved to travel and my parents, Mark and I had many holidays in America. Our sense of adventure came from my mum's side because there was no talk of them settling for a holiday in Scarborough or Blackpool. Instead, her extended family went to Sitges, twenty-odd miles outside Barcelona, almost every year. A Mediterranean break for a working-class family from Yorkshire must have seemed very exotic in the late 1960s – even if they didn't realise that Sitges was about to become one of the most popular tourist destinations for gay men in Europe.

Years later, Mum would tell us how it took them a week to travel from Castleford to Sitges in a small convoy of cars because, as well as her parents, Jimmy and Nancy, and her sister, Sue, they would be joined by her Auntie Audrey and Uncle Barry, their children and various other relatives and her grandmother, Emily. They drove down to Dover, took the ferry, and meandered slowly through France before reaching Spain. The days blurred as they stopped at any French roadside they fancied and camped for the night. They ate instant mash out of a packet, tinned soup and baguettes as they couldn't afford to go out for meals. The ground they slept on was rock hard as they also didn't have any air beds – but they loved it.

They would spend a week in Sitges and then take another week to travel back. A fortnight of driving, for a week in Sitges, seemed a fair exchange for such a colourful family.

My life became much more routine. I no longer had a boyfriend and, as an A-level student, I kept my head down. Sixth-form college felt like a big jump and I was now working alongside bright academic kids from across the region. I had to graft hard to keep up with the best students and get the grades I needed for university. Most of my spare time was taken up with revision and Mum used to urge me, without much success, to go out more and take a break from the books.

I would not be distracted, even when we went on holiday to America. My parents saved hard and we had a fantastic trip to the Florida Gulf Coast. But I still insisted on taking my textbooks so that I could revise every evening. Mum was horrified – and not just because it meant our luggage was close to being overweight. She couldn't believe that I also said I would have to come back five days early, on my own, so that I could study properly at home. But Mum and Dad knew how much it meant to me and so they reluctantly agreed that I could leave the holiday before them.

It paid off and, in the summer of 2001, I got the A-level grades I needed to get into my top two university choices, Manchester and Sheffield. As I wanted to move further afield and become more independent I settled on Manchester as my dream start to a future career in physiotherapy.

*

I still missed Rob, but we were no longer in contact. It was easier for me not to follow his rugby career and so I was only vaguely aware that Rob had made his first team debut for Leeds when he came on as a substitute against Hull in April 2001. He was chosen to start the following week, and scored Leeds' only try in a heavy defeat against Warrington. Rob showed great promise and defied all those doubters who said he was far too small to ever make it as a pro rugby player. He captained England's U-18 squad on a tour of Australia and New Zealand and by October 2001, in my first month as a university student, he was named as Super League's Young Player of the Year. Rob had turned nineteen a few weeks earlier on 26 September 2001.

In our contrasting ways we were defying all those who'd said we would never make it in our chosen fields.

I was excited to be at university but the first day of my course was disconcerting. When we got into the room the woman lecturer said to our class of female students: 'Right, strip down to your bra and your knickers.' I thought: *Oh, my goodness. What have I signed up for?*

But of course it was early confirmation that our course would be very practical, and hands-on, and as soon as we put on our medical gowns and began learning how to treat various injuries, the embarrassment melted away. From then on, I wore my best underwear whenever we were due our next practical session.

I stayed in halls at uni for my first year. I enjoyed myself, but I again put work ahead of my social life. I wasn't seeing anyone and, although I had a good group of friends, I kept the partying to a minimum. I probably missed out a lot on the social side, but physiotherapy was a demanding course. While some students had as little as one or two lectures a day, in physio we were in five days a week, pretty much from 9 to 5. The exception was Wednesday afternoon, which was reserved for sporting activities, but the rest of the time was occupied by a highly structured programme. We also had to do numerous clinical placements in six-week blocks, so it felt like we were at university to work.

I had a successful first year and, when we picked up again in October 2002, I was keen to do even better on my course. For that second year I moved into student accommodation with four other girls, three of whom were also physios but planning to specialise in different areas to me. After I'd settled in to our new flat in Manchester I was sitting on the bed in my room one evening when my phone beeped. I looked down and saw a text message.

I felt my heart skip when Rob's name shone on my screen. I was surprised but thrilled.

It was always a real source of regret how we had finished and I was sure my chance with Rob had gone. I had thought: *Okay, lesson learned. You won't do that again.*

So I was stunned to hear from Rob. I didn't know what to expect as I opened his message but, as soon as I started reading his words, I could hear Rob's voice in my head. He was lovely as ever, asking how I was enjoying uni and saying that he often thought of me. But I could tell that he was also sad as he explained that his grandmother was very poorly. It sounded like she did not have long to live. I knew how much Rob loved his family, and he adored his grandparents, and so I felt touched that he had contacted me when he was feeling so low.

We exchanged a few texts and I tried to console Rob. I felt our old closeness in those tender messages.

It did not take much longer for Rob to say how much he missed me. He wondered if there was a chance we could get back together again.

I could have played it cool – and I later joked with Rob that I should have made him suffer a bit more after he had refused to answer my texts or take my calls when I'd tried to patch us back together two years before. But as soon as I read the question, I knew the answer.

I replied immediately with an enthusiastic 'Yes!' I think I made it very clear that I would love to go out with him again because my phone pinged soon afterwards and Rob, who seemed very excited, asked if he could give me a call.

Once we had spoken, I felt even more certain, and we agreed to see each other that weekend. I had a Saturday job at Next in Castleford and Rob said he would pick me up in the evening and we would go to the movies – just as we had done when we were fifteen. But, this time, we wouldn't be on a double date with Glenn and Kim, and I was pretty sure that Rob would not be drowning inside a leather jacket that could have belonged to his dad.

Instead, Rob looked very flashy when he arrived in a bright red Toyota MR2 sports car. I was more impressed by the fact that he was so gentle and thoughtful. He went out of his way to make me feel special and I forgot that we were in a glitzy car as we chatted away happily.

Rob had booked tickets for us to see *Serendipity* – a romcom set in New York and starring John Cusack and Kate Beckinsale who bump into each other for the first time in Bloomingdales. They look perfect together, naturally, but decide to leave it to fate as to whether they will meet again. Of course bad luck keeps getting in the way, and they are kept apart and start different lives with ill-matched partners. But it's obvious that they will meet again, fall in love and end up together. It was a bit cheesy but Rob and I both smiled when the inevitable happy ending finally happened. Just before the credits rolled we watched them kiss, outside Bloomingdales, on their first anniversary – eleven years after first meeting.

It was a typical Hollywood movie, but it suited us perfectly that Saturday evening in Leeds. As Rob held my hand, and we walked back to his car, I felt happier than I had been in a very long time. I just knew we were right together.

I remembered how my dad once said that he had only one piece of advice to offer when it came to my love life: 'Marry a tall man – and bring some tall genes into the family.'

I was in no rush, but I would happily ignore my dad's joke.

I had never been more sure of anything in my life. Rob Burrow, standing five foot five inches tall, was the one.

4

The Wisdom of the Mad Giraffe

We feel drained and exhausted after the emotional earthquake of the last four days. Yesterday had been taken over by Jackson's party and so we needed today to be low-key. It's been a day of quiet recovery. We just took the kids swimming and then to the park before we watched a movie with them at home. After getting them off to bed early, Rob and I now sit close together in the front room of our new house as we watch the BBC's Sports Personality of the Year Award.

I am hoping it will be a mindless distraction but we are soon swept away by a strong and surging undercurrent of meaning for us personally. We see the sporting memories of a year that has just been turned upside down. As the montage of sporting footage clicks through the months, we can't help but reflect on how different our own world had looked, compared to now, in January or April, June or September.

The programme also takes a hushed pause away from the dazzle and applause as photographs are shown of sportsmen and -women who have died over the past twelve months. We stare in silence but I know Rob is asking himself the same question that I am: Will he still be here a year from now? We both desperately want to believe he will – but how can we forget that the consultant said Rob's life expectancy had been reduced to less than two years?

It seems even more heart-wrenching when, just before Ben Stokes is celebrated as the Sports Personality of the Year, they announce the recipient of the Helen Rollason Award for 'outstanding achievement in the face of adversity'. Helen was the first female presenter of the BBC's old Saturday-afternoon sports programme *Grandstand*. She died in 1999, having been diagnosed with cancer two years earlier, but she faced her illness with admirable resolve. Helen also helped raise more than £5 million, which was used to build a specialist cancer wing at the North Middlesex Hospital, where she received most of her treatment.

Each year, the award in her name is given to a person who has overcome the obstacles of their serious illness or disability with perseverance and courage and gone on to excel in sport or life. I feel choked up when this year's winner is named as Doddie Weir, the former Scotland rugby player who was diagnosed with MND two years ago. I've never heard of Doddie before but thoughts of MND consume me now. Rob admits that, as he hardly follows rugby union, he too has only a faint awareness of Doddie's past sporting achievements. But we are transfixed now because Doddie is receiving the award 'for raising awareness of motor neurone disease through his charitable foundation'.

The programme is being broadcast live from Aberdeen and it's deeply moving to see the giant figure of Doddie, all six foot six of him, walk slowly to the stage in his yellow-and-blue-checked tartan suit to the sound of bagpipes playing 'Flower of Scotland'. When he finally reaches the stage he smiles shyly and then has to bend down awkwardly, like a tall giraffe on spindly legs, as he politely kisses the cheeks of Gabby Logan and Clare Balding.

Princess Anne prepares to make the presentation. She is obviously fond of Doddie and, after praising him for his past excellence on the rugby field, says: 'I've been a patron of the Scottish MND Association for over thirty years and I know what a difference you've made to the understanding of motor neurone disease, its impact and your ability to fund research.'

She looks up at Doddie towering above her. 'For *that*,' she continues, placing a special emphasis on his contribution to fighting MND, 'we're all extremely grateful. It has been a real pleasure.'

Princess Anne, a surprise winner of the BBC Sports Personality of the Year Award in 1971 as a horsewoman who specialised in eventing, turns to the audience after the rapturous applause dies away. 'I have to say he was nearly a competitor of mine,' she says, 'but they couldn't find a pony big enough for him.'

Doddie chuckles awkwardly and I warm to him even more. 'Doddie,' she says. 'It's a real pleasure to give you the Helen Rollason Award.'

My heart cracks a little as Doddie says, 'Thank you, thank

you', his words slurring in that trademark sign of advancing MND.

Doddie is encouraged to say a few words. I remember all my past conversations with MND patients who struggled with their speech and imagine the difficulties for this gentle giant as he prepares to talk in public and on national television.

But all my misgivings melt away as, with a twinkle in his eye and confidence in his voice, Doddie speaks. The slurring doesn't matter because the words fall so sincerely from his mouth. 'Ma'am, thank you for your kind support, not only for Scottish rugby but with MND,' he says to Princess Anne before looking out at the teeming crowd of sporting celebrities. 'BBC, thank you very much for this most amazing award.'

I look in wonder at Doddie's wife and their three teenage sons. They gaze at Doddie with such pride.

His smile grows even wider as he says: 'It's quite ironic being a Scottish rugby player in the nineties because this is the closest I ever got to a trophy.'

Laughter fills the auditorium and I glance at Rob. His face is wreathed in a lovely grin as he stares at the tartan colossus who carries the same deadly disease as him. I can tell how much he already admires Doddie.

'To win a trophy is absolutely outstanding,' Doddie says. 'What a great Christmas present this has been, to show awareness of MND ... I've been involved in sport for a long time and what it does show [you] is [whether] you have a bit of spirit and fight. And my fight is to find a cure for MND.'

I notice how Rob leans forward as he looks intently at Doddie. 'With that,' the big man says, 'I have to dedicate this lovely Helen Rollason Award to everybody who has supported my foundation over the last two years. It's been truly amazing. I would not be standing here if it wasn't for the lovely support. The generosity has been staggering and my foundation has been able to pledge nearly five million pounds in trying to beat MND.'

The applause rises to a crescendo and my eyes shine in appreciation of the mighty Doddie. I want to stand up and applaud him too, but I dare not break Rob's concentration as he listens so carefully.

'The other thing that rugby and sport has taught me,' Doddie suggests when silence finally returns, 'is to enjoy oneself. Enjoy the day because we don't know what happens tomorrow. So tonight will be a pretty special one . . .'

He can't stop himself from laughing, as if he is thinking of all the riotous nights he has revelled in years before. The audience join him and I am astonished to see so many happy faces and hear so much laughter surrounding a presentation devoted to MND.

'In finishing,' Doddie says, 'I would just like to thank everyone but, most importantly, my family, my boys, for supporting me . . .'

Doddie's voice cracks over these last two words as, suddenly, he is locked in a fight to choke back the tears. One of his sons begins to cry as his mum looks up proudly at him. They join his two brothers, and the thousands of people watching, in applauding this open-hearted display of love. There is pain, too, as the massive figure of Doddie looks down, willing himself to regain his composure when he must have wanted to howl with anguish. The sustained clapping helps and Doddie soon appears calm and strong again.

'Ladies and gentlemen, always leave the best to thank to last. That's not you Hoggy, that's not you Gaz, that's not you Kenny Logan or Robbie Wainwright. Sorry. It's for my good and lovely wife, Kathy. Thank you so much.'

The camera pans across to Kathy who looks beautiful and almost serene as she smiles at Doddie. So many emotions churn through me, but, for the first time in almost eighty hours since Rob's diagnosis, I feel a sense of lightness – hope even. It's obvious how happy and close the Weirs are as a family. Their pride in each other fills the arena and resonates from the television screen. I see Kathy draw in a deep breath as her beloved husband continues praising her.

'Your support has been amazing. Your strength and patience has been outstanding – because I know I'm not the best patient. But you get on with things. You feed two people, you dress two people. Thank you very much.'

I see the future for Rob and me in these intimate moments. A time will soon come when Rob won't be able to pull on his socks, underwear and clothes or tie his shoelaces. He will not even be able to spoon food into his mouth, let alone walk or talk. But rather than terrifying or traumatising me, I feel sure that Rob and I will be as one, just like Doddie and Kathy.

The standing ovation would rumble on for a long time but Doddie, knowing that the BBC has a show to complete, shouts:

'Thank you very much for the lovely support. Have a good night and a good Christmas.'

I'm not sure whether to laugh or to cry but Rob knows what to do. He turns to me and beams. 'What a man.'

Gabby Logan, whose husband, Kenny, had been part of that earlier joke, agrees as she hails 'a true inspiration, the 2019 Helen Rollason Award recipient . . . *Doddie Weir!*'

Doddie has to crouch down a long way so he can kiss Gabby's forehead as he thanks her again. Then the face of another famous Scottish sportsman fills the screen. Rob knows I haven't got a clue who it is, so he explains that Chris Hoy, a track sprint cyclist, has won six Olympic gold medals. Hoy's eyes swim with tears but steely admiration and respect are embedded in his features.

Rob and I feel the emotional depth and power of Doddie's appearance even more acutely. We watch the rest of the show in a daze, not really talking about all we have seen. It's clear that we will discuss everything soon but, for now, with the children tucked up in bed, we simply look at the athletes glowing with health. Rob will chip in every now and then to identify someone I don't know but, for the most part, we watch in stunned, companionable silence.

In the past I would have chattered through the programme or flicked through my phone. Tonight is different. It really does feel like the start of the rest of our utterly changed lives. Doddie and Kathy have made such a difference. Rob and I are not alone.

*

The following morning I felt like giving Rob Burrow my annual Father of the Year award yet again. It was typical of Rob that he insisted on taking Macy and Maya to school. They were about to start the last week of term and he was determined that the best way to protect the children would be by retaining a sense of normality. Most of us would just want to curl up and hide away from the world after receiving the kind of shattering news that had rocked Rob to the core. But he refused to surrender to despair.

Rob knew we needed to keep going and so he smiled and teased the girls as we chivvied them to move a little quicker as they got ready for school. They had no idea about MND or what it meant and so, on a cold winter morning, it was the usual domestic rush to find their tights and shoes, pack their school bags and lunchboxes and check that they hadn't forgotten anything. Rob made sure we stayed on track while holding little Jackson in his arms.

Christmas was coming and we faced the horrible challenge of picking the right time to explain to the children that their dad would soon need special care. Trying to find the right words, so that we were honest but avoided frightening or upsetting them, would be one of the hardest but most important things we would ever have to do. Our focus for the weekend had been Jackson's birthday but, once Monday morning rolled around, it was plain that we could not put off that painful conversation much longer. While they were at school we would decide the next steps.

The girls loved the fact that Rob took them to school every

day. Few other dads did the same and yet it had always been Rob's way. Even when they were very small, he took them to many of their pre-school playgroups. I can't think of many other men, let alone Super League rugby players, who were happy to be the only dad in a room full of mums and kids as they all sang 'The Wheels on the Bus' together. Of course, there were times, as a player or coach, when rugby training ran over into the afternoon and Rob could not get away. But he always did his best to juggle his schedule or come home straight after training so that he could be with the children. There were a couple of playgroups where some of the mums were convinced that Rob, who was so chatty with everyone, was a single parent. That's why he was my constant Dad of the Year.

Rob had very solid and perhaps even old-fashioned family values, which were handed down to him by his mum and dad. Politeness and respect for others were fundamental principles for him, while putting the children and me first was at the heart of everything Rob did. He instilled that sense of decency and kindness into Macy, Maya and Jackson and tried his best to always be completely involved in their lives. It meant they adored him and that life with their dad was not just confined to an hour before bedtime or on the weekends – as it understandably has to be for so many working parents in more regimented jobs.

Our children were fortunate to have a mum and a dad who were around so much – only for fate to intervene in such a cruel way. But we resolved to keep the harsh reality hidden from them for a little while longer.

Apart from our parents and siblings we had only told a few very close friends about Rob's health. We had, of course, shared the news with Angela, and Rob had confided in Barrie McDermott, Kevin Sinfield and a few other former teammates at the Leeds Rhinos. We knew we would have to open up to more people, but at that time everything seemed overwhelming.

When Rob returned from the school drop-off he agreed to stay at home while Jackson had a nap and I nipped into town to get some essentials. It was the first time I had been alone since that terrible Thursday afternoon and I drove into Pontefract in a kind of trance.

I parked the car and walked to the cashpoint on the corner of Ropergate, one of the main streets running through the heart of Pontefract. I was operating on automatic pilot as I took my bank card out of my wallet and slotted it into the cash machine. The screen clicked into gear and requested my PIN. My right hand stretched out to the metal keypad and then . . . I stopped. I didn't know what to do next. My brain had frozen.

I forced myself to breathe in deeply. It was not that difficult. All I had to do was type in the four-digit number that I'd used thousands of times before. But my mind was blank. I could not remember a single digit of my code. It was as if I had been stricken by dementia. My hand hovered uselessly over the screen until, eventually, my planned transaction was cancelled. My card slid out of the slot and back towards me in cold rebuke.

I wondered if I should try again in the hope that my memory would return second time around. But two people were queuing behind me and so, bereft and humiliated, I put the card back in my wallet and turned away from the cashpoint. I must have looked distressed because the woman waiting behind me smiled sympathetically. I walked away hurriedly, just wanting to get home.

I walked through the front door, almost relieved that I still remembered where we lived, and then burst into tears as soon as I saw Rob. I explained what had happened and he reassured me that my mini brain-fade was to be expected after all we had been through. Then Rob squeezed my hand and said, 'I'm sorry, darling.'

It was my turn to comfort him and point out that he no had reason to apologise for an illness that was beyond his control. I promised him that I'd be okay and that my brain would click back into gear. But, first, we needed to work out when we told the kids.

'We'll do it later today, after school,' Rob said with sudden certainty.

His assurance bolstered me. We decided I would speak first to the girls' school as it was important that they understood how Macy and Maya's home life was about to be affected. I knew we were doing the right thing because our delayed conversation with the kids had been hanging over me. It felt as if we were hiding the truth from them. Rob and I believed that if we told them now they would soon be distracted by the excitement of Christmas, which might help soften the jarring news of their dad.

Jackson, having just turned one, was obviously too young to be included in our chat. Maya was only four, but she was bright and perceptive. Macy, at the age of eight, already showed real emotional intelligence. I knew she would pick up on our distress if we didn't talk to her.

As I waited to get through to the school, I felt myself trying to control waves of panic and doubt. Would I be able to cope with looking after Rob, Macy, Maya and Jackson on my own? Was I strong enough? Who might I turn to for professional support if I needed it? Should I be thinking of finding a counsellor for the children? Would I be able to help them find a way through the pain of their dad's terminal disease? How could I comfort them when the inevitable happened and they lost their dad for ever?

These were understandable and legitimate questions. But, years later, I have learned enough about trauma and bereavement to address such fears. I've also spoken to plenty of wise people – one of whom pointed out that children tend to 'puddle jump'. They will jump in a puddle and be sad because their feet are suddenly wet and muddy. But then, a minute later, they'll jump straight out of the puddle and feel happy because their boots have made a ridiculously squelchy sound. In contrast, an adult will jump in a puddle and get stuck in the depressing mud. Children are much more resilient than we think and they can move quickly from one emotion to another. When it comes to living in the moment they are much better than we are.

I also now understand that it is healthy and truthful for them to know when you are upset. I used to think that I had to always look unbreakably strong for the children. But now I know that if they see me break down and cry it helps them understand their own hurt and grief. If I can cry, they know they can definitely shed as many tears as they need to. They would also learn that admitting vulnerability and sadness is actually a sign of a deeper inward strength.

I still had many lessons to learn, however, and Mrs Carr, the assistant head teacher at the school, helped me hugely when I called to explain our changed situation. She was kind and calm and made some telling points when I asked her how best I might talk to Macy and Maya about illness and death. She said that, when the unthinkable happened and Rob died, it was important that I did not attempt to hide the truth. I should not say 'Daddy's gone to sleep' or 'Daddy's gone to a better place.' If they heard those words they might become frightened of going to sleep themselves in case death came for them. And by talking of 'a better place' I would be implying that our home and their love had not been enough for Rob. In more extreme cases it could provide a disturbing link with suicidal thoughts and a child might think, *I want to escape and go to that better place*. It was best to be honest while helping the children to feel loved and supported – and reassuring them that there would still be so much fun and happiness in our lives together.

I felt so much better after talking to Mrs Carr. That evening, soon after they had demolished their tea, Rob and I sat down with Macy and Maya. We spoke as sensitively and thoughtfully as we could. The girls listened quietly and then Maya piped up, saying: 'Why are you telling us all this? It's boring. Can we watch some TV?'

We couldn't help but laugh. Her innocence, delivered with the blunt honesty of a child, wiped away our anxiety and dread.

I hugged her tight, and Macy too, and allowed them to turn on the television. Rob and I had a real chuckle as we chided ourselves for getting so worked up about telling the kids.

'We've just got to try and relax and live normally,' Rob reminded me. 'Worrying endlessly is not going to help any of us.'

Macy, being four years older than Maya, absorbed the news in a different way. She didn't say much at first but, later, she came to find me with a serious question. 'Mum,' she said, her eyes full of concern, 'is Daddy going to die?'

She was right to ask and I tried to give her the answer she deserved. We sat down and I explained that her dad's disease was serious and that, yes, he would eventually die. But I stressed with real clarity that Rob and I believed that this would not happen for many years. Her dad was a really determined person and he would do all he could to look after himself.

'And Daddy's got us, hasn't he?' I said. 'We'll take special care of him, won't we?'

Macy smiled, giving me a sudden burst of sunshine. 'We will, Mum,' she said. 'We really will.'

I learned in later years that Barrie had asked Rob, before his diagnosis, if he suspected he might have MND. It emerged that Rob was more worried than I'd known, but he had tried to brush away the concern of his friend. When Barrie asked him to meet for a coffee, before the medical tests were done, Rob had been typically late. In their usual jokey way, Barrie had tapped his watch and said: 'Come on, dickhead, you're later than normal!'

But when Barrie became serious he asked Rob directly about the slurring in his speech. Rob blamed it on stress but Barrie felt a deeper trepidation. He understood the gravity of MND because the wife of his friend had the disease. Rob, however, shook his head. 'It's not MND,' he told Barrie. 'I'm fine. Don't worry.'

Kevin Sinfield had confronted Rob even earlier. In September, two months before his diagnosis, Kev had asked Rob about his slurring: 'You've not had ten pints tonight, have you?' It was a joke because Kev knew that Rob didn't drink. But it was the prelude to Kev, who was effectively Rob's boss as the director of rugby at Leeds, calling a meeting. Rob worked as the head Academy coach and he couldn't avoid a formal conversation in Kev's office.

'Look, Rob, what's going on?' Kev asked. 'I'm worried about you.'

Rob eventually admitted that he was dealing with stress and struggling with his old shoulder injury. But he told Kev that he was keeping the painkillers under control and that he was sure the slur in his speech would soon disappear.

Kev wouldn't let it go, however. He insisted that Rob see the team doctor to talk about his shoulder and the slurring. That decision led to the consultation and the tests; during that time, Rob admitted to Kev that he had been googling symptoms of MND. So they had all been mightily relieved when the consultant ruled out that possibility after Rob's MRI scan came back clear of any brain anomalies.

But their darkest fears were about to be confirmed.

On the Thursday evening of 12 December, Kev kept checking his phone. Finally, at around half six, hours after Rob and I had heard the catastrophic news, Kev sent a text. He asked Rob how the consultation had been.

Rob was still reeling and his reply was brief: *I've got MND. It's been confirmed.* Kev was devastated after he had turned to the internet to discover the gravity of the disease.

He was closer to Barrie but it still took Rob another full day to send a longer text to him. *I've got motor neurone disease. I don't know how long I've got but I'm going to give it a good crack. Don't worry.*

Barrie admitted that he had 'sobbed uncontrollably' at home. He was so distraught that his wife, Jenny, had to comfort their teenage children – they were convinced that there had been a death in the family. When Barrie could finally talk to them he explained how much Rob meant to him and how vital it was that they kept the news to themselves.

He met Rob at their favourite Starbucks the following afternoon and Barrie conveyed, with all his vast empathy and friendship, that he was ready to support us no matter what lay ahead.

Kev and Rob also talked over a coffee. Their conversation had such an impact on Kev that, unknown to Rob and me, he contacted Bryan Redpath, a close friend of Doddie Weir. Bryan, another former Scotland international, had been Kev's coach at Yorkshire Carnegie, where Kev had played rugby union for a brief spell after he left the Rhinos. Kev had asked Bryan if Doddie might consider meeting Rob.

Everything moved quickly and I was startled when Rob told me on Monday evening that he and Kev were going to drive up to Carlisle on Wednesday afternoon to meet Doddie. Rob clearly needed the meeting, but I hesitated when he suggested we watch the new documentary about Doddie and MND. I was worried that we would both be pulled down by something so raw and revealing.

But Rob knew better than me and, a few hours later, we were both uplifted and hopeful after watching *One More Try* – an immensely moving documentary. I was heartened to see Doddie still working a little on his farm in the Scottish Borders and to feel the warmth and love between him and his family. There was so much fight and hope in Doddie, which we wanted to match.

Rob was very nervous when Kev picked him up early on Wednesday afternoon. They were due to meet Doddie and Bryan at the Holiday Inn in Carlisle at six that evening and a normal two-and-a-half-hour journey could take much longer if they hit traffic. But they got lucky and arrived well before five. Rob's nerves worsened while they waited.

But then everything changed once Doddie turned up. He arrived with Gary Armstrong, yet another Scottish international who now doubled as his informal driver. Bryan was with them too but there was no need for him and Kev to make any introductions. Doddie took charge and his friendly good cheer and openness settled Rob immediately.

Doddie began by laying out some of the simple lessons of life that MND had taught him. He now valued life – and all the people that mattered most to him – more than he had ever done before. The experience of living, for Doddie, seemed heightened in its intensity. The pleasures of life, which he had once taken for granted, now felt rare and almost exquisite. He was determined to squeeze every last ounce of fun and joy out of each new day.

Doddie did not try to sanitise the harsh truth of MND. He told Rob about his deterioration and how helplessly dependent he had become on Kathy. There was no attempt to sugar-coat the reality that death and the future of his family was often on his mind.

They knew little about each other's code of rugby – beyond that they were physical and brutal games. Doddie reminded Rob that they had both taken some almighty hits and been knocked to the ground, but still they'd got up. They'd fought on and found ways to outwit a tougher opponent, whether that was a dazzling sidestep or an ankle-tap on an 18-stone prop for Rob or a sneaky punch in a ruck or early jump at a lineout for Doddie.

They could do the same and leave a mark on MND.

In the end they would probably lose, but they could still celebrate small victories along the way – whether it was wearing slip-on shoes when you could no longer tie your shoelaces, or changing the channel on the remote without asking for help. Both those simple tasks were now beyond Doddie, but he had bigger challenges in mind. He was far from done.

Doddie made Rob laugh as he showed him how to use a

variety of aids that helped him eat, walk, sit and even drink a beer out of an adapted pint glass. Most of all, Doddie encouraged Rob not to surrender to the ravages of the disease.

'Give the old bastard this,' Doddie said as he stuck two fingers defiantly in the air.

At the time, Doddie's consultants were trying to persuade him to have a feeding PEG (percutaneous endoscopic gastrostomy) fitted as it had become a battle to swallow. But Doddie had refused the PEG. For him, acceptance would feel like he was surrendering to the disease. So he would keep going, even when Kathy eventually had to feed him nothing but puréed mush with a spoon. He would still be flashing those two fingers at MND.

Doddie explained, as they all laughed, that his old teammates called him the Mad Giraffe. He liked it and the crazy madness meant that he would keep on defying the cold hard logic of MND. He was dressed in his trademark yellow tartan 'troosers' and the jokes began to flow because the three stocky little scrum halves – Rob, Bryan and Gary – were as quick with the wisecracks as they had once been when slipping through a gap in the opposition.

But there was also a striking compassion, and even wisdom, in the Mad Giraffe. He reassured Rob that he was going to be okay with our special family and a strong group of friends in rugby. We'd all rally round him and, because they were well-known former players, Doddie and Rob would always have great public support.

Doddie was more worried about the postman and bricklayer, the farmer and fireman, who had to face the same savage disease on their own. He spoke about his foundation – My Name'5 Doddie (he replaced the letter S with the number he had worn as a lock forward). He explained that not only were they trying to raise millions to help researchers find a cure, but Doddie wanted to help ordinary men and women who were much more anonymous and alone than him and Rob. He also wanted to tackle the government and force them to take MND more seriously and commit much more meaningful funding to fighting the disease.

When the time came to say goodbye, Doddie made sure Rob understood that it would only be a fleeting farewell. He was ready to see Rob whenever he needed advice, a boost or just a good old moan. Rob had his number; he just had to hit the button on his phone and Doddie would be there to talk to him. Rob was genuinely moved by such generosity but he was soon laughing again when Bryan showed him the photograph he had taken. Doddie was a foot and an inch taller than Rob but, on Bryan's phone, the height difference looked even more comical.

The Mad Giraffe gave him a wink. 'You're going to be all right, wee man,' he told Rob. 'I can tell.'

Rob had gone into the meeting like a blind man trying to feel his way through the desolate darkness. Everything was so new and so bleak that he'd felt lost and helpless. But Doddie helped him to see again. Doddie helped turn on the light.

But the quiet elation Rob had felt in Doddie's company faded on the long journey home. After he and Kev had spoken for almost an hour about the inspirational lessons Doddie had shared, they fell into a contemplative silence. It was raining hard, in a persistent winter deluge on a bleak December night, and the windscreen wipers worked at full speed.

Kev imagined how he would feel if he was in Rob's unfortunate position, already in the grip of MND and facing a terrifyingly uncertain future. He would be anxious about the consequences for his wife, Jayne, and their two teenage sons. What would Kev need to help him and his family cross such treacherous terrain? How much support would he need before he knew that Jayne and the boys would be safe after he was gone?

Slowly and gently, Kev began to ask Rob about his deepest fears. Rob was intensely proud but he conceded that thoughts of leaving me and the children haunted him. He was wracked with guilt and dread.

'I know,' Kev said. 'I would be the same. But listen, Rob, you've got me and some real mates. We'll raise some money. How much do you need?'

Rob shook his head in the rainy dark. 'No, Kev,' he said. 'I'll work something out.'

Kev, who already knew that Rob would never work again, persisted.

'We'll be all right,' Rob said. 'Lindsey works.'

But Rob – and Kev – knew that my life would soon be dominated by caring for him and so Kev repeated himself. 'How much do you need?'

It was a tough but necessary question and Rob tried to evade it. Kev knew how much Rob was earning at the Rhinos, at the age of thirty-seven, and so, with urgency, he said: 'Let's work it out now.'

They began to talk properly then and it did not take long for them to calculate what Rob needed in the immediate future. Kev said the figure out loud.

Rob began to cry but, through the tears, he nodded. Kev was also crying but he didn't dare look again at Rob.

The rain lashed down but they had a plan. So they drove on through the drenching darkness, silent amid the tears and the soft screech of the wipers whirring against the glass, back and forth, back and forth.

5

Two Worlds

'Hey up, big nose!' Rob shouted at Barrie McDermott as he walked into an otherwise empty dressing room. 'You must have told some lies in your time, Pinocchio.'

It was five o'clock on a late-summer afternoon in 2004. The two and a half hours before kick-off stretched ahead of the small scrum half and massive prop forward at Headingley, home of the Leeds Rhinos. Rob, having had seven espressos and three Red Bulls over the course of the long wait of game day, was wired. His friend, teammate and mentor greeted him with a wry smile.

'You've shown up at last, big mouth,' Barrie said.

Rob grinned as he was on a roll with his insults. 'Next time you pick a nose, Baz,' he suggested, 'pick a smaller one.'

Barrie looked down at his wise-cracking pal and muttered: 'So says Rob Burrow, the only man with a life-size image of himself on his passport.'

It was hard for Barrie to pretend that he was grumpy for too long and they both laughed. They were always the first two players to reach the ground, often an hour before the bulk of the first-team squad turned up, and they loved the familiar pattern. Barrie lived just outside Oldham and it could often take an hour for him to drive to Headingley. He worried about the traffic on the M62 and so it was far better, and more relaxing, to arrive early.

Rob could make the journey from our new home in Pontefract in forty minutes, but he followed Barrie's lead and left soon after 4:15pm for a 7:30pm start. He parked in the same spot every week because he was superstitious and nervous. Rob needed that time with Barrie before their teammates arrived. It didn't matter who they were playing, or how well Rob had performed in the previous game, because he would say the same words over and over again.

'Are you nervous?' he always asked Barrie. 'I am. What about you, big schnozz?'

'You're making me nervous with all your yapping,' Barrie growled.

'It's a big game, Baz,' Rob said, talking fast, as he always did whenever he was anxious. 'So are you nervous?'

'Just don't fuck it up like you did last week. You're the reason we nearly lost.'

Barrie was smiling but he knew that the shift in Rob had started. The comic jibes were over, at least for a while, and Rob's insecurities were about to come flooding out. There was a ten-year gap between them and Rob was still in his early twenties, while Barrie had already played over 300 games in Super League. He had made more than 250 appearances for the Rhinos and, before then, played forty games for Oldham and thirteen for Wigan. Barrie was also an established international.

Rob was still in the formative stages of his career but that pre-match apprehension, and those doubts, would never leave him. Years later, in his final season in 2017, when he had played 200 more games for Leeds than Barrie had, Rob would still turn to other players for reassurance. But from 2001 to 2005 he relied mostly on Barrie to bolster him.

Barrie understood that all the talk of nerves and doubts were part of the ritual for Rob. His little pal was one of the most competitive and mentally tough players he had ever met. Once they left the sanctuary of the dressing room and stepped into the furnace of a brutal and testing Super League game, Rob played with a delicate mix of audacity and conviction.

His courage ran so deep that commentators often said he was fearless, as he chopped down yet another giant brute of an opponent by taking him low and hard in the tackle, with exemplary timing and technique. And he exasperated rivals by slashing through their defence as if they were hardly there. He had so much speed and trickery that his diminutive size and low centre of gravity became a kind of superpower. When the opposition threatened to gang-tackle him, in an overwhelming show of force over brilliance, the Rhinos shielded him. They looked after Rob because he meant so much to the team and to them as people.

But before he was consumed by the heat of battle Rob needed Barrie to calm and encourage him. The prop reminded Rob how much they would depend on and help each other. It was important that Rob should tell Barrie whether the next pass was coming his way. Rob needed to tell other key players the same thing so that they would all be expecting the ball – and then it was up to Rob to decide who was best equipped to power them forward.

It was a reminder to Rob that, as their number 7, he really was in control and yet supported by his tough teammates. Whenever Barrie conveyed this same simple message it was as if Rob absorbed it afresh, for the very first time.

They made an unlikely partnership, but their bond was strong. Barrie took the brunt of Rob's wisecracks, but he was there for his friend when they needed to talk seriously about rugby and life. In the dressing room, with the game only hours away, Barrie listened patiently as Rob wondered if he was ready. Was he good enough? Was he sharp enough? Was he smart enough?

Barrie reassured him again and again. He pointed out how well Rob had done all season, with some Man of the Match performances, and how he had blistering pace, not to mention a devastating side-step, which left so many of their opponents for dead. Speed meant so much in the modern game and Rob had more than anyone in Super League. Barrie reminded Rob that, pound-for-pound, he was the strongest member of the team, with more stamina than any of them.

Whenever they did the bleep tests the proof was clear. Rob was the quickest Rhino; only Mark Calderwood, on the wing, gave him a real run. And when it came to the endurance tests Rob led the way. Kevin Sinfield would give everything of himself and be left in agony on the ground after it was all over. Not only did Rob do better than Kev, he made it look easy.

But still, that game day (and every game day), Rob remained nervous and uncertain. Barrie put the black humour to one side and spoke even more firmly to Rob, reminding him of their excellent training together all week in the two-man drills. He pointed out that he'd chosen Rob as his partner because, despite the difference in size, the scrum half pushed him harder than anyone.

Barrie believed that training in an elite environment was not necessarily about getting a win every day. Sometimes you had to put yourself in a situation where you would lose, while gaining so much more from the lessons you learned. A few times every week Barrie would set up a small grid, 5 x 5 metres, and say: 'Right, Rob, I want you to try and beat me with your footwork and agility. If you do it nine times, I'll try and make sure I catch you the next time.'

After Rob zipped around him for the tenth straight time, Barrie reduced the space of the drill to 4 × 4 metres. When that didn't help he cut it down to 3 × 3 metres, saying: 'C'mon, Rob, give me a chance here.' Rob, with his fast-twitch fibres, was so quick and elusive. For many other speedsters in rugby league, their pace decreased when they changed direction. Rob was different. When he veered away from a despairing dive he actually increased his speed because there was such power and spring in his muscles.

Barrie told Rob how similar he was to the great Jason Robinson, the rugby league wizard who had switched codes to union and helped England win the World Cup in 2003. Within five steps Rob and Jason were close to top pace and then could maintain that speed while swerving in, out and away from opposition tackles.

It had been that way since Rob's debut season in 2001. At first, when he was invited to train with the first team, Rob had looked all teeth, nose and ears to Barrie. There was hardly anything else to him because he was so tiny for a rugby league player. Barrie had played against the five-foot-five Alfie Langer, the revered Australian who had signed for the Warrington Wolves in 2000. But Langer was much chunkier than Rob and looked stronger.

None of that mattered. Most players were six feet tall, weighing around 100kg, but Rob ripped up the template. He had been surprising people in rugby league his whole life.

When he first made the senior squad, Rob was remarkably quiet and shy. But it did not take long for him to run rings around the rest of them, both on and off the field. Barrie always said he would prefer tackling a six-foot-four monster than a cheeky little devil like Rob.

He was full of even more devilment off the field. No one else enjoyed farting as much as Rob did among the groaning Rhinos – but he was very different with me and treated me as a princess who lived in a fart-free realm. At Leeds, in contrast, Rob would be chased by all those glowering and furious teammates who were the butt of his jokes and pranks. He was sneaky and smart, and full of schoolboy stunts.

As he was often the first off the training field Rob would rifle through his friends' bags in search of their keys or underpants. If he found a player's keys he would hide them or, if he had enough time, actually slip out to drive the car to another location. His underwear tricks were even more juvenile. Teammates would howl when they returned to the changing room to discover that their smalls had been left sodden in the shower or smeared with chocolate on the inside to leave the most infuriating of fake skid marks.

On other occasions, and much to my shock and embarrassment hearing these stories long after Rob had retired, he would causally pee on a teammate standing next to him in the showers. As a battered and weary player washed his face or hair, with eyes closed beneath the cascading water, he had no idea Rob was adding to the deluge. Only the yelps of amusement from the others alerted the victim to the fact that Rob was weeing on him.

There were a few times when Rob looked close to being murdered by a teammate who put him in a headlock. But Rob either escaped or the aggrieved Rhino let him loose; they all knew him so well and loved him despite the toilet humour and maddening wind-ups.

Rob was canny too because he never played such tricks on Barrie or captain Kevin Sinfield. They both warned him that their revenge would know no bounds and Rob was wise enough to believe them. He chose his targets carefully and, when it came to Barrie, he made sure that his attacks were merely verbal. But there was a method to his madness.

In choosing Barrie (and in later years the giant New Zealand prop Kylie Leuluai) as his prime victim for a verbal roasting, Rob sent a message to all the other Rhinos that he really was fearless. Going after the biggest men proved that it did not matter that he was by far the smallest member of the squad. Rob knew that Barrie and Kylie were too kind to ever hurt him, but everyone had to stay on their toes around him.

By the time Kev arrived in the dressing room before a game, the anxiety of the Leeds number 7 had been mostly curbed by Barrie's reassurance. Rob still asked the same 'Are you nervous?' question of Kev, but he would need much less of a pep talk compared to the one he'd had from Barrie. Kev would offer precise reminders of why they worked well together. Rob had been twelve and Kev fourteen when they'd first met at the Academy, and they'd developed so much alongside each other in the subsequent years.

Kev and Rob were not close friends then but the respect and admiration they had for each other was vast. And so, buoyed by Baz and Kev, Rob always found a new calm just before the game.

He'd reach for his headphones and, in moments as sacred as they were inspirational, Rob would listen to the speech Al Pacino gave, as a grizzled old football coach, to his team in the film *Any Given Sunday*. Rob had an incredible memory and could reel off word-perfect chunks of dialogue from *The Office* or any of the countless Hollywood movies he loved.

Rob knew the Pacino speech off by heart too. Occasionally, he would mimic the opening and, in a gravel-voiced and pretty unconvincing American accent, walk around the dressing room

in nothing but his shorts and say: 'Three minutes to the biggest battle of our professional lives . . . it all comes down to
today. Either we heal as a team or we're gonna crumble. Inch
by inch, play by play, 'til we're finished.'

Most of the time, however, the speech meant so much to
Rob that he listened to it in silence before running on to the
field. Through his earphones Rob heard Pacino say: 'You know,
when you get old in life, things get taken from you . . . But you
only learn that when you start losing stuff.'

In the movie, the team listening to their old coach begin to
stir, murmur their appreciation or say, 'Hell, yeah.' As Rob
looked around at the Rhinos, lost in their individual forms
of preparation, Pacino's words resounded.

Barrie watched Rob walk slowly around the dressing room,
immersed in the intensity. He looked as serene as he was determined, as inspired as he was committed. There were no more
questions about nerves as he listened to the culmination of a
favourite movie scene.

'You gotta look at the guy next to you. Look into his eyes.
Now, I think you're going to see a guy who will go that inch
with you. You're going to see a guy who will sacrifice himself
for this team because he knows, when it comes down to it,
you're gonna do the same for him.'

Rob removed his headphones and tucked them away in his
bag. At 7:15, as everyone else switched off their mood-setting
playlists or go-to songs, the room became hushed and concentrated. When Kev and Barrie walked around to give specific
messages to individual players, they left Rob alone. It was only

near the very end, just before they walked down the tunnel, that Barrie looked across at him.

Rob nodded at his protective friend. He was suddenly free of nerves and doubts. He was all set to light up the game with his electrifying pace and thunderous courage. He was ready.

I knew so little about Rob's world of rugby and only began to really understand what he went through, and how much he achieved, when talking years later to Barrie McDermott, Kevin Sinfield, Danny McGuire and Jamie Jones-Buchanan. When Rob and I moved in together he was emphatic that he didn't want to live in Leeds; it was important that he drew a clear distinction between work and home. As soon as he walked through the front door he seemed to forget all about rugby and never wanted to talk about training or playing. I heard nothing about his high jinks in the dressing room or his insecurities before games.

In the same way, Rob would never gloat about his achievements or celebrate the tries he scored or the big wins he and the Rhinos racked up with impressive consistency. He would be the same man I loved when we were out, even when wide-eyed fans came over to congratulate him or to ask for an autograph or photograph. Rob was always polite and friendly but I could see how relieved he was when it was just the two of us again.

He seemed happiest at home with me. As soon as training was over or a post-match briefing ended, Rob would jump in his car and drive back to Pontefract. His teammates were surprised at first because most players, even the non-drinkers, liked going out as a group. The Rhinos hardly ever persuaded Rob to join them, but because they all loved him and accepted his ways, no one gave him a hard time about preferring to be with me rather than them.

Rob learned to be a little more careful after he had a nasty accident in his beloved bright red MR2 with its personalised number plate. The Rhinos used to do savage training sessions at Roundhay Park in Leeds, where the coaches would flog them with punishing drills up a steep hill. Rob did better than everyone else and, true to form, he was always the first out of the car park and on his way back home.

Barrie and Kev used to drive to training and back home together every day from near Oldham and, a few minutes after Rob, they pulled out of the car park. They hadn't gone very far when they turned a corner and were shocked to see a car on its side.

'Shit,' Kev exclaimed, 'that's Rob car.'

'There he is,' Barrie shouted, pointing to the surreal sight of Rob climbing out of the window of his overturned MR2.

Rob had skidded and flipped on the icy surface before crashing into a giant oak tree. The car and the poor old tree were both badly dented but Rob, much to everyone's huge relief, was unscathed. Once they had made sure he was all right, Baz and Kev teased him about his Hollywood escape. But it was time for him to become a little less cavalier.

Rob had enough money to put a deposit down and pay the mortgage on the house we bought in Pontefract. Until I qualified and began working as an NHS physio at the Leeds

Teaching Hospitals Trust, my financial contributions were limited by the small salary I earned from my Saturday job at Next. But I made up for it in other ways.

When he first moved away from his parents, Rob was pretty hopeless. He couldn't cook or clean and he still took all his washing home to his mum. Rob also didn't know how to pay a bill, let alone set up a standing order, and he left everything to his mum to sort out. So when I finished uni and moved in permanently with Rob, I took over the running of the house.

It worked because we complemented each other so well. I was organised and practical while Rob was laidback. He was always on time while I was often late. I made detailed plans for the future while Rob was content to play video games and watch comedy shows and movies. I studied hard while Rob liked mucking around.

We once went to Dubai on holiday at the same time as Barrie, his wife, Jenny, and their three children. When Rob heard that the McDermotts were off to a water park he wanted us to join them. So, while I sat under an umbrella with Barrie and Jenny, and they allowed me to get on with my studies for my next physio exam, Rob flew down the slides with the kids. It was a good day for all of us.

Rob still drove me mad sometimes. I drew up sensible lists for the weekly supermarket shop but Rob would casually buy multiple wicker baskets from the QVC shopping channel. We had no need for even one wicker basket but it set a pattern. So I wasn't totally surprised that, one day, Rob bought us a robot vacuum cleaner – even though he never used our old Hoover himself.

After we got engaged at Disneyland in Paris, Rob became even more scattergun in his purchases. I came home from a long day of work in Leeds and was startled to see that locks had been fitted to the garage door. When I asked Rob what had happened, thinking that perhaps we had been burgled, he said a young guy had knocked on the door that afternoon. He was selling locks and, as it was obvious that he'd not had much luck all day, Rob took pity on him and bought a small collection. We didn't need any locks but that was typical of Rob.

But we were similar in other ways. We both wanted to succeed in our careers and look after each other. We loved going to the movies or out for a meal. If there is such a thing as soulmates, I'd like to think it was us. We were two halves of a whole. We were opposites who became a perfect match.

Rob's career was soaring – even if he kept seeking reassurance from Barrie before each game. Barrie just marvelled at the quality and passion of Rob's play.

They regarded St Helens away as one of their hardest games of the season but, one year, Rob shredded the Saints and scored two tries. He soon raced away for another try. Rob was ecstatic with his hat-trick – only for it to be chalked off by the video referee. It turned out that, much earlier in the move, Barrie hadn't touched the ball with his foot.

'I'll never forgive you for that, big nose,' Rob fumed. 'If you'd done your job and played the ball properly, I'd have had a hat-trick at Saints away.'

Barrie just grinned and shrugged: he understood the competitive fire that burned in Rob. He had scored two great tries and was desperate for a third. Rob was furious – for about five minutes after the game. By the time the team bus arrived back in Leeds, he'd accepted Baz's cheerful hug of apology with a smile and jumped in the car to drive home. Rob never mentioned his fleeting disappointment to me. The moment he walked through our door he was attentive and loving.

In 2004, Rob helped the Rhinos end a 32-year-wait for the Championship as they beat Bradford Bulls 16–8 in the Grand Final. The following season he was in scintillating form and he made twenty-nine starts in his thirty-four appearances for the Rhinos, scoring twenty-one tries, as the same two teams again contested the Grand Final. This time, victory went to the Bulls 15–6.

Rob made his international debut on 29 October 2005, when he played for Great Britain against New Zealand at Loftus Road in London. He was on the way to somewhere very special in rugby.

I had also found my path in physiotherapy. After qualifying I did my junior rotation, gaining valuable experience working in critical care, neurology and respiratory care of the elderly. I eventually decided to specialise in musculoskeletal physiotherapy, which focuses on muscles, joints, posture and movement with patients after surgery, injury or illness.

After I successfully achieved my Band 6 post, which is a level of grading expertise in physiotherapy, I needed to make a choice. My next logical progression would have been Band 7 in musculoskeletal physio, but this kind of work was divided in two. A proportion of my time would be devoted to clinical work while the remainder required a managerial role. I was far more interested in pursuing the clinical route and moving away from management. I decided to jump grades to Band 8 so that I could work alongside a neurosurgeon and an orthopaedic spinal surgeon. My specialisation in spinal pathologies and injuries was challenging and stimulating with years of learning ahead of me.

But first, in 2006, the year Rob and I both turned twenty-four, we had a wedding to plan.

Saturday 30 December 2006, St John the Evangelist Church, Ripon, North Yorkshire

A winter wedding suits Rob's rugby schedule best of all. But there is also something romantic about getting married on a cold but beautifully sunlit afternoon in Yorkshire. The old church looks gorgeous as I take Dad's arm and he leads me down the aisle. Rob and his best man, Kevin Till, his oldest friend, are in the front pew. They turn around with everyone else to look at me.

I wear a ruched and strapless white wedding dress with a full-length cloaked veil that drapes discreetly over the A-line skirt. My hands are tucked away and kept warm in a white muff. It feels as if my heart is racing but Rob settles me as his smile grows the closer I come to him. He stretches out his left hand to take my right arm as we stand before the vicar – who makes a little joke about it being 'time for kick-off'. I force myself to laugh even though a fresh wave of nerves washes through me.

We sing 'Silent Night', and then there is a Bible reading, before the vicar talks about our marriage and the new world we are about to build together. Snatches of his sermon stay in my head as he discusses building a house and a family. He mentions my grandmother Nancy as being one of fourteen and says that Rob and I both come from strong families. The vicar says how important it is that our house of love should be built on a rock because – as if he can see into the future – he suggests there will be a storm ahead. But the house will stand firm if it is built on a rock of belief. He promises that when life becomes hard, God will be there for us – offering strength and comfort in good times and bad times.

When it is time to exchange our vows, I remove the muff. The familiar old words ring out, made different by the fact that our names are now bound together. 'Robert,' the vicar asks, 'will you take Lindsey to be your wife?'

Rob, without a moment's hesitation, says: 'I will.'

The vicar turns to me to ask the same question: 'Lindsey, will you take Robert to be your husband? Will you love him, comfort him, honour and protect him, and forsaking all others be faithful to him as long as you both shall live?'

My voice is clear: 'I will.'

The vicar turns to address the congregation. 'Will you,' he asks, 'the families and friends of Lindsey and Robert, support and uphold them in their marriage now and in the years to come?'

There is a unified chorus: 'We will.'

After a brief prayer the vicar grimaces. 'It's time for a forward pass,' he says. 'It's the worst sentence in the whole of our liturgy. Who gives this woman to be married to this man?'

My dad steps forward and says: 'I do.' He takes my hand so that Rob can now hold it.

The vicar chips in again. 'And he doesn't sound relieved. Right, here we go.'

Rob echoes each line the vicar says to him and then it is my turn to repeat the vow. I make this solemn promise:

> *'I, Lindsey, take you, Robert, to be my husband,*
> *To have and to hold*
> *From this day forward.'*

Rob smiles at me with almost unbearable tenderness. He knows how much I mean every word:

> *'For better, for worse,*
> *For richer, for poorer,*
> *In sickness and in health,*
> *To love and to cherish,*
> *Till death us do part.'*

After we exchange rings, the vicar says: 'I proclaim that they are husband and wife.'

I could burst with happiness as Rob is told: 'You may kiss the bride.'

Applause resounds through the church. After we sign the register the vicar hands over the certificate and makes another of his little jokes. 'Don't lose it,' he tells Rob. 'You'll need it for your old age pension.'

Rob and I just want to get outside now; as he relaxes, he slips his right arm through mine and his left hand into his pocket.

We laugh when, in the wintry sunshine, we're showered in confetti by our whooping friends and family.

In the car, a silver Rolls-Royce with a number plate that reads W88DNG, my voice sings out. I sound very young, even to me, as I say: 'I was so nervous.'

Rob just sounds thrilled. 'Amazing,' he says. 'I loved every minute of it.'

As the driver turns to us, Rob grins in delight and introduces me: 'This is Mrs Burrow now.'

When we walk into our reception at Oulton Hall Hotel near Rothwell, I get called by my new name for a second time when Kevin, as best man, shouts: 'Please be upstanding for Mr and Mrs Burrow . . .'

Rob and I can't stop smiling through the meal and then the speeches. My dad speaks first and while joking about me, after saying that we have made him and Mum very proud, the whole room erupts in laughter. Without meaning anything intimate, Dad says, 'Rob always put a spark into Lindsey.' I blush, my dad looks confused and Rob makes an amused cutting gesture with his hand. But it's soon Rob's turn to look embarrassed; he takes a swig from a bottle of beer as my dad mentions his rugby achievements.

Rob smiles more easily again when my dad, standing between me and Mum, turns to him: 'Rob, me and Sharon couldn't be any happier that you've married our daughter, Lindsey, and we are very proud and honoured to have you as a son-in-law. I'd like to wish you both health and happiness all your lives.'

Dad then leads a toast and it only feels a little strange to see everyone raise their glasses to us as they say, in unison, 'Lindsey and Rob.'

Rob takes the mic next and cracks an early joke about his height as he wonders whether he should stand on the table so that everyone can see him at the back. But, spotting Barrie, Rob has more fun with the big old Rhino. After saying how he hoped we had all enjoyed the delicious meal Rob points at Baz. 'On the off chance that there's some leftover food, there's a big fat bastard at the back, waiting in anticipation of it. Sit down, Barrie!'

Baz, who knows more about Rob than most people, gives a regal wave.

Rob is at his most moving when he speaks sincerely. The room is hushed as he pauses. 'Most importantly, I'd like to say a few words about my wife, my Princess Lindsey.'

As if we are suddenly alone, Rob shakes his head in wonder and says: 'Wow, darling. You're absolutely beautiful.

You really are. I can't believe that a girl like you would ever want to marry somebody like me. I stand here pinching myself that somebody as special and gorgeous as Lindsey could walk into my life. I mean that, Lindsey. Do you know, I'm actually going to spend the rest of my days together with you?'

I would be embarrassed if I didn't feel like welling up as Rob keeps talking. 'I'm honestly so proud to have found you, Lindsey, I really am. I firmly believe that you don't marry somebody you can live with. You marry the person you cannot live without, and that's certainly the case with you, Lindsey.'

Rob suddenly grins as if remembering everyone else in the room. 'I'm the soppy one,' he says. 'It seems me and Lindsey have known each other for a lifetime. She certainly was my high-school sweetheart, back in the day when we were about fifteen. I dreamt that she would one day be sat here at my side as I give this speech to her as my wife. So I'm really chuffed now.'

After he tells a few stories about our past and my appalling lack of rugby knowledge Rob returns to how he truly feels: 'Honestly, jokes aside, I've been trying to tell you in words what Lindsey means to me. It would take a lifetime to try and show you. She's an actual princess and all I can say is I'll give her my all, the best in my life, I really will.'

Looking directly at me again Rob says: 'Lindsey, we can have as many years together as our parents have done – and many more. I'd like to make a toast to the most beautiful girl in the world, my wife, Lindsey Burrow. If you'd all be upstanding. Lindsey Burrow.'

After I've been toasted again by everyone Rob says: 'In finishing, I would just like to say, darling, I'll give you the best life I can and I promise to never let you down. I'd like to stay with you, and grow old along with you, because the best is yet to be. Thank you for making me the happiest lad in the world.'

The room rocks with cheering and applause – as it does again during Kevin's speech. 'Me and Rob have been through a lot in our lives,' he says as he explains that he had asked his best friend what he wants from marriage. 'Rob replied: "I want to be a model husband" – which is fine. "I want to be a model citizen." Yes, we know he's that. "And I want to be a model lover." So, being a bit curious about his answer, I decided to look up the word "model". In the dictionary it says: "Model: a small, miniature version." '

As people hoot with laughter, Rob laps it up, as he does when Kevin speaks warmly of me. But it's my turn to glow with pride when Kevin describes Rob as being, despite his great rugby career, 'the most down-to-earth and genuine guy I know'.

We have tried to make it a special wedding and Kevin explains that we've set up a chocolate fondue fountain and a casino in the Rothwell suite. Everybody looks ready to party, but it's time for Rob and me to take to the dancefloor for our first dance as a married couple.

We've chosen to strut our stuff to '(I've Had) The Time of My Life' by Bill Medley and Jennifer Warnes. It comes from the finale of *Dirty Dancing* – although Rob knows that I used to think they were singing about Noah's Ark rather than the hottest time of their lives. That's just my thing, which I picked up from Grandad Bully: getting the words to songs totally wrong.

Neither Rob nor I are very good dancers, but all his competitive juices were flowing once we began practising months earlier. We worked so hard for so long. It meant a lot to us because, after all, it was at Noreen's Dance School that I danced with his sisters and met Rob.

As we take to the dancefloor Rob looks as ready as he does when walking out of the Headingley dressing room before a big game. He is about to become Patrick Swayze to my Jennifer Grey.

The music starts and, as we glide across the floor, I look at Rob in surprise and horror. They're playing a different version of the song to the one we know so well. 'It's okay, Linds,' Rob says as, channelling his inner Al Pacino in *Any Given Sunday*, he grabs me by the hand. 'It's still the same song. I'm with you. I've got you. We can do this, darling.'

We can and we do. It's not perfect and we miss the big show-stopping lift but I still feel great as Rob keeps talking to me all through the dance, counting out our steps while checking our feet and keeping me on track. We go for a big twirl, his arm around my waist while I hold him gently around the neck. Then, holding hands, we shimmy towards our audience.

Everyone is clapping in time and roaring us on. Rob still looks really concentrated. I love him all the more as he urges me: 'Keep going, darling! One more time!'

I keep dancing, smiling at my husband, feeling like the luckiest girl in the world.

6

Opening Up in Lockdown

Rob will be home soon and I need to see him. I need to know that he has got through this long and painful day with his spirit intact. Waiting for more news has been hard, but at least the children are content. They've had their tea and Macy and Maya are watching something on the iPad while Jackson is happily crawling around in the front room with me. I can hear the chatter of the girls upstairs and it helps.

A couple of days have passed since we told them about Rob having MND and they have been as bright and cheerful as always. After our important second conversation, when she asked me if her dad was going to die, Macy has been typically lovely. Maya takes her cue from her big sister and, with both of them feeling reassured that they are safe and loved, she has made me laugh and want to keep cuddling her. They also have an inexhaustible energy, which keeps the house humming. But there is no swimming tonight, as Christmas is coming, and so the hum is peaceful.

Jackson is oblivious to everything outside his secure little world. He is curious about how it feels to push himself up and stand, a touch unsteadily, before he takes a few steps that end with him falling down on to his cushioned nappy. Jackson laughs – just as he does when his dad lifts him up high. Rob loves to carry Jackson around on his shoulders and I'm relieved that he hasn't stopped.

I remember how we felt at this time exactly a week ago. Last Thursday, in the deep darkness of a December evening, we were reeling from the diagnosis. I was on my way to swimming with the girls while Rob sat in shock with his parents and sisters. We had no idea then how we would piece together our shattered lives.

But we are stronger and more positive now. On a scale of 1 to 10, where the lowest mark matches the devastation of last Thursday and the highest score takes us back to our blissful days before MND, I might have moved up to a 3. It's not great but the difference between now and last week feels profound.

Doddie Weir gave us our turning point and, most of all, the hope that it was possible to live a good life despite MND. Last night, after meeting Doddie in Carlisle, Rob looked transformed. Doddie was diagnosed with MND in December 2016, when the specialist predicted he would no longer be able to walk the following Christmas. But, three years on, Doddie still has a snap to his step.

Doddie sets the example we will follow. We will accept the diagnosis but we will fight the prognosis. We will not hide from the fact that Rob has MND, and that his life expectancy and quality of life will be drastically reduced, but we're not going to curl up and hide. We will try our best each and every day that we have left together.

Rob was almost exhilarated after the Carlisle meeting. Apart from sharing Doddie's tips on how best to cope with the disease, he bubbled over with stories of how they had laughed. Doddie also spoke about his foundation and how they are raising money for research into finding a cure. He is determined to change MND's landscape of gloom and to bring doctors and patients, scientists and politicians into the same room. They will tackle the disease in positive and proactive ways.

I know that these are just aims, which will take years to implement, but they lift a weight from my shoulders. Last night Rob's eyes shone with belief and his hope became our hope.

Rob said he would listen to the advice of the doctors but he was going to prove them wrong. He would defy their prediction that he would live for just another year, or two at the most.

It makes me love Rob even more. Of course I know the inevitable outcome. But I will support him to the hilt and try to rise above the bleak reality of his condition.

'And Lindsey,' Rob said last night, looking at me intently, 'we need to have no more tears.'

I looked into his pale blue eyes and nodded.

'That's going to be our policy from now on, darling,' he said. 'No more tears. We've had our tears, and we needed them, but it will do us no good to keep on having them. It will be no good for the kids if we mope around, crying all the time.'

I struck a deal with Rob. We would keep those helpless tears at bay.

Rob knew I meant it, so he held me close and told me again that it was going to be all right.

He then surprised me when he said that he would go public with the news.

I soon understood. Rob wants to be as open as Doddie and help other people suffering with MND. Most of them don't have a friend like Kevin Sinfield who can just magic up a meeting with Doddie. So it's the right thing for Rob to tell the world that he, too, has MND.

This is where he is today. After he spoke to the Rhinos and Phil Daly, the club's head of media, an interview was set up with Tanya Arnold of the BBC.

Rob trusts Tanya because she has interviewed him many times after matches. But those were sporting interviews and, usually, Rob had just helped the Rhinos win another big game. This is different. This is Rob telling the world he has been struck down by an incurable disease.

A few hours ago I had a text from Rob. He said the interview was hard but that Kev helped him. He would speak to other people around the club, as he wants to keep coaching, and then drive home.

I look at the time on my phone. Rob will be back soon. I switch on the television as his interview is on the BBC's local news channel. The national news programme is almost over. I sit and wait, smiling as Jackson shows me a toy.

Now, with a jolt, it's very real. I hear my husband's name on the television.

Leeds Rhinos rugby legend Rob Burrow has motor neurone disease.

I want to cover my mouth in fresh shock at hearing this raw truth from a serious but immaculate newsreader on the gleaming box in a corner of our front room. Jackson doesn't understand a word and, instead of following the news about his dad, my little boy bangs his toy on the floor.

Rob sits between two framed photographs of rugby league glory at a room in Headingley. The patch of bare wall behind his head is painted in a shade so neutral that I can't even tell what colour it is meant to be. I am used to seeing Rob on television. He is usually covered in a light sheen of sweat a few minutes after a game. Not now. He seems nervous, in his Rhinos top and jacket, and it looks as if he is carrying a heavy load.

Silently, I urge Rob on. I know he will get through this and find the words. But it's so hard.

Tanya asks Rob when he first noticed signs that something was wrong. 'Um,' Rob says hesitantly, knowing that he is about to go down a dark and uncertain track from which there will be no turning back. But then, gathering himself, he starts talking. 'Probably a few months back. The family were telling me I'm slurring my speech a bit, which I was. Being a little short-tongued, I never really took notice or believed them. Then at the point I was seeing the doc for my shoulder, an old injury, I told him about my speech and from then it were really quick, three weeks, had tests and a neurologist, MRI. Just under three weeks, I got the results diagnosed. When I went to see the specialist, we were expecting to be told I had something which can be tret and move on, get on with your life.'

Rob has used that old Yorkshire word of 'tret' which means 'treated'. I want to smile, but for the fact that I'm hurting so badly for him.

'So when we went in the room and he told me I had it, [it was] a bit of a shock. Maybe it's the athlete in us all, where you don't want to lie down and just take it. I'm taking it as a challenge. I don't intend to lie down. I will get stuck into it and [it will be] a bit like my career.'

Tanya nods encouragingly and then says: 'It must be tough on your wife, though, and the kids.'

'Yeah,' Rob says, his slightly slurring voice now knotted with feeling. 'That's the emotional side.'

He glances to the side and the news editor cuts away to the adjoining photograph of Rob holding up the Super League trophy. But the camera is soon trained on Rob's face again as he continues. 'You know, I suppose you have your good days, your bad days. But, um . . .'

Rob manages to say 'yeah' before lowering his head. He breaks down then, the tears rising up from deep inside him. His body shakes as he tries to stifle his quiet crying.

It feels as if my heart is hammering inside my chest. Rob needs me but I know this happened hours ago and I wasn't there. I am torn already, wanting to be with Rob always, while wanting to be with the kids too at such a vulnerable point in our lives. My eyes swim as I stare at the screen, not knowing what to do, as I watch Rob crack open.

Tanya averts her gaze, with compassion, and Kev steps in. He walks across the room to find his little pal. Kev wraps his arms around him, his left hand cupping Rob's head while the right hand rests gently on Rob's back. Above the muffled sobbing, I hear Kev speaking tenderly: 'A couple of deep breaths. You're doing great.'

Instinctively, Rob has reached out to Kev. I watch as, from another camera angle, we see Rob's left hand pat Kev on the back. It's the same pat Rob has given me whenever we've hugged over the past week.

After the screen turns black for a moment, Rob resumes talking to Tanya. 'I feel it's just one of them things,' Rob says in his gravelly voice. 'I'm unlucky and it just happened. I've tonnes of family support. My club and, in particular, Kev can't do enough for me.'

We are told that a crowdfunding page has been set up to help our family. I don't know what to think and Rob is swamped by emotion again. 'When people want to help you . . .' Rob says, his mouth crumpling. He soon lifts his head but it's a struggle for him to get the words out. But, somehow, he resumes his interrupted sentence.

'And you can't repay them. It's humbling, very overwhelming and [I'm] forever grateful. Can't thank them enough.'

The last image is of Rob looking straight at Tanya. It is pure Rob – open and loving, caring and thankful.

I mute the television and listen to the children, lost in their innocent worlds. I make the most of these moments to find the strength I am going to need in the coming hours, days, weeks, months and however many years we have left.

When Rob gets home, I tell him, with genuine belief, how well he has done today.

Rob has good news of his own. Everyone at the club has been great and they are keen for him to keep coaching. We will be able to keep life as normal as possible for a while longer. Rob also shows me the message that Doddie posted on social media:

> I met with @Rob7Burrow last night and offered him whatever help and support he might need at what is a difficult time for him. Meeting another sportsman suffering from MND has strengthened my resolve to help find a solution to this condition.

We spend the next few hours putting the kids to bed, having a meal together, and then trawling through the thousands of messages that have flooded Rob's Twitter page. Rob writes a short message of thanks:

> Today has been a big day for me and my family but I would like you all to know I have read every message and post. I can't explain how overwhelmed I am at the reaction I have had from people throughout our amazing sport. Thank you so much, from the bottom of my heart!

The tweet carries the time, date and our location: *8:39pm. 19 Dec 2019 from Pontefract, England.*

This is a significant moment because everything has changed. The world now knows what we are facing. It feels strange because, throughout Rob's career, we have been intensely private. We are happiest in the company of each other, and our family.

But we are less lonely now than at any other time this past week. We hope that someone else who has MND, or who is caring for a loved one with the disease, might feel less alone too. We can't take away anyone's despair or isolation, but maybe Rob can make a small difference.

Our first Christmas with the disease passed in a numbed haze. The children were excited and happy, which was all that mattered, and Rob and I held it together. We spent the day at my parents and then went to see Geoff and Irene and everyone else. Presents were swapped, masses of food was laid out, jokes were cracked, and we all avoided saying those dreadful three letters together. We didn't mention MND over Christmas and New Year.

A new decade, the sparkling 2020s, did not offer us a fresh start. It forced us down a harsh path. But, oh, the kindness we received as the new year began was extraordinary.

Soon after Rob's diagnosis in December I had been phoned by Claire Lang, the clinical nurse assigned to our MND team. Claire was our first point of contact before meeting the various clinicians and consultants who would look after Rob. She was lovely but she spoke honestly. Claire said that, early in January, we would meet Dr Agam Jung, our neurologist. Claire warned me to steel myself and Rob. She told us that Dr Jung could be very matter-of-fact and direct. But this was her way of cutting through the niceties so that she could speak clearly about the issues we faced. We should not make the mistake of thinking she was abrupt. Instead, we would learn that she was an exceptional doctor.

I worked closely with surgeons every week in my work as a physiotherapist so I was used to blunt medical talk. We would just appreciate hearing Dr Jung's candid views on how best we could manage the illness. I didn't tell Claire that Rob was also intent on proving every doctor wrong as he was determined to live for so many more years than they predicted.

But when the moment came to enter Dr Jung's office at the Leeds General Infirmary, I felt a tremor of trepidation. I knew how fragile both Rob and I were and I worried that an unforgiving prognosis might crush us. I took in a deep breath.

It was not needed. Dr Jung swept us away with her kindness and warmth. She was a beautiful and smiley Indian woman who had been working in the UK since she'd arrived for neurological training in 2004. Dr Jung told Rob she considered it an honour to look after him.

After discussing Rob's condition, Dr Jung suggested that our future meetings should be held at Seacroft Hospital in Leeds. She had developed 'a one-stop shop' for her MND patients so that they could have all their needs attended to in a single visit to her multi-disciplinary team. Apart from seeing her we would also be able to meet a speech and language therapist, an occupational therapist, a physiotherapist, a psychologist and more practical technical staff who'd help us with a wheelchair and other appliances we might need.

Dr Jung didn't make any false promises or give any dire warnings. Instead she spoke calmly and empathetically. She also explained that she was not involved in any research studies that might, one day, find a cure for MND. It was more important for her to work in the here and now and help her patients feel better. This made so much sense to me as I realised that MND would not be cured in Rob's lifetime. It seemed more helpful to know that Dr Jung would pour all her considerable expertise into making Rob comfortable.

Dr Jung had a terrific sense of humour, which meant she and Rob clicked straightaway. I felt all the tension drain out of me as she and Rob swapped wisecracks. Living with MND would be bearable with Dr Jung on our side.

She urged us to keep working closely with the speech therapist who had already been to the house. It was vital that everything was in place when Rob's speech deteriorated so much that we would battle to understand him. Neither the speech therapist nor Dr Jung could predict how many more months Rob would be able to talk coherently, but new technology could help him retain a voice.

A speech app would allow Rob to communicate by typing out a text, which could then be broadcast as an audio message. A company called SpeakUnique could replicate Rob's accent and intonation so that it would sound as if he was saying the words out loud. The alternative was to use the standard metallic voice, which had become synonymous with Professor

Stephen Hawking, the theoretical physicist who had lived with a slow-progressing form of MND for fifty-five years.

It took decades for Hawking's paralysis and complete loss of speech to emerge. Rob's strand of MND was very different. It was aggressive and fast-moving.

Rob grinned at the idea that he might end up with an 'American robot voice'. He was more enthused by the encouragement of Dr Jung and the speech therapist to 'bank' his voice by reading a short book out loud so that the technology could emulate his vocal pitch and delivery.

I think Rob might have been, initially, a bit offended that, on her next visit to us, the speech therapist brought over *The Tale of Peter Rabbit* for him to read. He might not have been too comfortable reading about quantum physics in Stephen Hawking's *A Brief History of Time*, but a children's book seemed to indicate that she did not have a high opinion of the literacy level in rugby league.

We soon learned that the recording device just needed a few hundred simple words to be stored by Rob and the technology would do the rest. I liked the fact that we had a practical plan; again, I was blown away by Rob. He might have preferred to read the script to *The Office* or Al Pacino's speech in *Any Given Sunday*. But he picked up *Peter Rabbit* and read it aloud with a winning mix of seriousness and wry humour.

The next step into the public domain for Rob, now a warrior against MND, came a few days later. On Wednesday 8 January 2020, he spoke to reporters at Headingley about his unlikely return to the field with the Rhinos. That Sunday, Rob would play the last few minutes of a friendly against the Bradford Bulls.

The purpose of the game was to celebrate the testimonial of Rob's great friend and former teammate Jamie Jones-Buchanan. It was typical of Jamie that he had decided to share the proceeds from the match with the fund that had been set up to help our family. In just a few weeks more than £200,000 had been raised. The generosity of strangers astonished Rob and me.

As a thank-you to Jamie and everyone else, Rob attended a press conference in the week of the game, where he spoke impressively about coping with the early stages of the illness. The previous day, Rob and I had been to Sheffield to see Professor Christopher McDermott, a neurologist who specialised in MND. Dr Jung supported the visit as Professor McDermott knew more than she did about research into the disease.

'Professor McDermott is a really top guy,' Rob told the press. 'He did confirm I have MND, but he reckoned I could be alive for a few years yet, which is good. He spoke about some trial drugs, so hopefully I'm eligible to get on that. That's really positive news.'

Rob also spoke about the kindness of people and picked out a few who had been in touch with him. 'The amount of support and messages that have come in is incredible. The best thing for me is not how they talk about me as a player, but how they talk about me as a person. That's the most humbling thing of all. You bring your kids up to be nice people and that's the most important thing – how people have spoken about my personality. It's absolutely unbelievable.

'The message from Wayne Rooney was humbling. He's one of the best footballers ever and for him to say something like that about me is incredible. I tweeted him directly afterwards thanking him. I couldn't believe he knew who I was, let alone him saying "Good luck." He replied by saying he loved watching me play and I couldn't believe that was real. I'm just a normal person who admires people like Wayne.

'The amount of people with MND who have got in touch, be they famous or not, is amazing. They've all told me their stories and I just want people to know that I've read all their messages and listened to their advice about what to do. I've had a lady in Miami get in touch to say she was diagnosed at thirty-seven and she's now fifty-six. And look at Stephen Hawking – he lived with it for years. I'm really positive and really determined. I'm not sure I'll win the battle but I want to be here for a long time. I want to watch my kids grow up, and my head space is really positive. The first couple of weeks were emotional but now I'm just getting on with it.'

It felt as if the old Rob was back and he spoke with relish about the prospect of sharing a dressing room one last time with Jamie, Kevin, Kylie Leuluai, Danny McGuire, Jamie Peacock and everyone else. 'To go on the pitch with some old friends will be really special. It's incredible to get out there, but I'll stick to two or three minutes. The whole point is about going on the pitch and playing for the club I love. The whole rugby family has got on board and I'm sure there will be fans of other clubs there on Sunday. The whole game epitomises the support I've had. Again, it's just overwhelming.'

At 4:46 that Sunday afternoon, 12 January, that emotion went into overdrive as Rob took the field to play the final ten minutes of the game which, remarkably for a pre-season friendly, was being screened live on Sky Sports. The stadium was sold out and the entire 20,000-strong crowd rose to salute Rob – just as they had done before the match when he walked out with Jackson in his arms and Macy and Maya alongside him. I felt so proud, if desperately sad as I knew the afternoon probably marked the last time that Rob would ever walk across a rugby pitch.

The score didn't matter – Leeds won 34–10 – compared to the fact that Rob was on the pitch with his friends. Keith Senior had retired nine years before in 2011, but he looked like a big kid as he grinned at Rob while they faced their old Bradford rivals, Stuart Fielden and Robbie Hunter-Paul, who had also dug out their boots for one last game. Supporters of different clubs from across rugby league had travelled to Leeds to say their own special goodbye to Rob. Bradford, meanwhile, donated their proceeds from the match to our family.

A beautiful afternoon was sealed when, at the end, Kev embraced Rob in a heartfelt hug and our kids joined their dad on the pitch.

'I was tired but I absolutely loved every minute of it,' Rob said at the press conference. 'I'm not one for the limelight but it's been a big day. After this . . . it's back to normal life. That's changing nappies and some coaching and the sooner I get back to that the better. But how can you not enjoy a day like today? In rugby league we stay together and look after our own. Today was an example of what our game is all about. You don't know how much it means. No words will come close to describing how I feel right now.'

Rob's smile was tangled. 'I've been struggling with my words anyway,' he said. 'I'm overwhelmed and humbled. Thank you so much.'

The world was about to change even more drastically. The whisper of a spreading virus in China turned into a deadly worldwide threat as, on 11 March 2020, the World Health Organization declared a global pandemic. The following evening we began to understand the gravity of coronavirus as the prime minister addressed the nation on television.

'This is the worst public health crisis for a generation,' Boris Johnson warned. 'Many more families are going to lose loved ones before their time.'

The language of the virus had already emerged and certain phrases, from 'self-isolation' to 'social distancing', were becoming familiar. But our full realisation that the world was about to shut down came on the sombre evening of Monday 23 March 2020.

'I must give the British people a very simple instruction,' Johnson said as Rob and I sat on the sofa, listening silently. 'You must stay at home. We must stop the disease spreading between households.'

People would only be allowed to leave their homes for 'very

limited purposes'. We could shop for basic essentials and take one form of outdoor exercise a day. Travelling to and from work, but only when it was absolutely necessary and could not be done from home, was permissible. Medical needs, or helping a vulnerable person, were also granted exemption from lockdown.

'These are the only reasons you should leave your home,' Johnson said. 'You should not be meeting friends. If your friends ask you to meet, you should say "No". You should not be meeting family members who do not live in your home.'

Rob and I glanced at each other. Our family is so important to us and we needed the support of Geoff and Irene, and my mum and dad, as we tried to adjust to the earthquake of MND. Our parents also needed to see us to make sure that we were coping. But we had to hunker down on our own, with the kids, in a cocoon.

'The way ahead is hard, and it is still true that many lives will sadly be lost,' the prime minister concluded. 'And yet it is also true that there is a clear way through.'

We would obey the legislation . . . but we were on our own. Rob and I would rely on each other to keep the children calm and sunny – and thankfully the weather helped in those early weeks.

In lockdown, one glorious day followed another and we made the most of the chance to be with Macy, Maya and Jackson. I was still apprehensive as we had no idea when we would next see our parents, but Rob persuaded me to cherish all we had. We spent brilliant days in the garden, playing with the kids. Rob was still a hands-on dad and he and the girls built obstacle courses for them to climb over. We also had noisy water fights and lots of barbecues.

At night we spoke to our parents on the phone and organised extended family quizzes and games on Zoom. There would be prizes for the winning team and we'd take it in turns to make up a goodie bag or buy some chocolate. It would then be dropped off outside the front door of the winners.

I remember lots of laughter in those first months of lockdown. It was only later that I understood that Rob had been struggling internally during some of our online get-togethers. He was usually the most quick-witted and funniest of us all, but while the quips flew back and forth, Rob was quieter than normal. I thought he was just tired but, in truth, he was floundering. He could think of rapier-like responses to all the wisecracks; but it felt impossible to turn the jokes he saw in his head into words we could all hear. His speech was fading fast.

The months passed. I noticed that Rob was losing weight and his movement was increasingly compromised. But he could still walk and, as lockdown rules eased slightly, drive us to parks further afield. We were also able to see both sets of parents, albeit sticking to the regulations as we stood ten feet away from them outside.

I could see how much Geoff and Irene wanted to hug Rob and it was hard to remind the children that they weren't allowed to be cuddled by their grandparents. But we knew how important it was to keep everyone safe. Each Thursday night, for many months, it was moving to open our front door at eight o'clock and join the nationwide applause for the NHS. The sound of clapping could be heard all the way up and down our street. It meant so much to me, a proud NHS worker for so many years.

We could not see Dr Jung or any of her team in person and I missed not being able to hear their assessment of Rob's condition. I knew he was deteriorating but it was hard to measure the extent – unless we were given obvious signals. We received one such jolt when Rob drove us across to Castleford to see my mum and dad for another socially distanced chat.

We were nearly there when, just before we took the last corner that turned into my parents' cul-de-sac, Rob lost control of the steering wheel and nearly crashed into a garden. He managed to press his right foot on the brake and we came to a shuddering halt just before he hit anything. Thankfully the kids thought it was funny and, even years later, they would recall the incident with some amusement.

Rob and I knew what it really meant and he didn't argue when I said I would drive the car up the road and on our return. Later, he nodded when I told him the truth: 'Rob, you can't drive again.'

When I called Irene to tell her the news, she immediately said that we had done the right thing. Rob's strength and dexterity were fading and we didn't want to put anyone at risk.

Glimmers of normal life returned. I worked from home, doing physio consultations on Zoom: the schools reopened and the girls returned to their lessons in masks. We also could have occasional visitors on the condition that we met outside, in our garden. It was a great boost to Rob as he loved seeing his close friends in person again.

Kev came across to Pontefract every two weeks. Barrie was another frequent visitor; sometimes he arranged for a few other Rhinos to join him and Rob as we could have up to six people in a socially distanced outdoor gathering. They shared so much laughter on those summer afternoons.

Rob had become even more lethal with his quips at their expense because he had begun to use the SpeakUnique app and text his words into verbal gags. MND gave Rob the liberty to be even more blunt than usual in his assessment of people they discussed. He was mostly generous, but he would occasionally call someone they knew 'a real dickhead' while gossiping with his pals. Barrie and Rob would laugh so much that there was only one thing louder than the sound of their cackling – and that was Rob's helpless farting. He couldn't control himself, or the strange noises rippling from his bum, as he rocked with laughter.

But they had plenty of serious conversations as they discussed the state of the game and the fact that some players across both codes of rugby had taken the legal route with their concussion cases. Rob, typing his words into the app, said: 'If playing rugby league has given me MND, then so be it. I would not swap it for anything.'

I knew it was true because, months earlier, Rob had told me he would never blame rugby for what had happened, and that he treasured his career more than ever. I found his words comforting because it meant that Rob was free of bitterness and resentment.

When lockdown became less draconian, Rob and I were approached by *BBC Breakfast* and asked if we would consider making a documentary about his first year of living with MND. Six months earlier I would have said an emphatic no. Rob knew this because, after their December 2019 interview, Tanya Arnold had asked him whether he thought I might talk to her.

'Lindsey?' Rob had said in disbelief, knowing me so well. 'You'll have no chance.'

Everything felt different in the summer of 2020. After the onset of MND, and then Covid, my perspective on life had changed. I had also learnt that 5,000 people in the UK were then fighting their lonely and quietly personal battles with MND. Rob felt an increasing responsibility to use his platform in rugby to bring the attention of the world to the disease.

We had also been reassured by the sensitive and compassionate way in which the *BBC Breakfast* team had covered Rob's story. When we met Claire Ryan, the producer, and Sally Nugent, the presenter, our minds were quickly made up. We forged such a bond with Claire and Sally that they soon became friends.

We allowed them into our home and to film us when we met Dr Jung. Even when we discussed with her the delicate matter of whether Rob would allow the fitting of a feeding PEG, before his throat muscles withered into near paralysis, we gave the BBC crew permission to film. We all wore masks and, though it was hard for Rob to make himself understood, I explained to Dr Jung that he wanted to resist using the PEG. Rob saw it as a surrender to MND.

Rob spoke well on camera, stressing 'my mind is so strong and positive'. I was less stoical and failed the no-tears policy, breaking down while describing the day of Rob's diagnosis.

But there were so many happy memories too as the film showed old footage of Rob as a tiny boy zipping past much bigger kids with his prodigious talent on the rugby field. Footage of his most famous moments in Grand Finals were interspersed with interviews and contrasting scenes from our current lives. Viewers saw me lift Rob up the stairs and the kids dance around him with silvery balloons on his thirty-eighth birthday on 26 September 2020.

The documentary was beautifully crafted and ended with Sally interviewing Rob in our garden. They sat in chairs placed ten feet apart. Rob used his app to type out his answers, which emerged in a computerised version of his voice.

'I am determined to beat this disease and it starts with a strong mindset,' Rob said.

He looked up from his phone, his dark glasses shielding his eyes from the sunshine, as he listened to Sally's reply: 'You certainly have that, Rob. You are an inspiration to us all.'

Rob smiled and, slowly, lifted his left thumb. Sally gave him a two-thumb salute and blew a kiss across the social distance. It was a gorgeous moment from our Covid times.

When Rob and I watched the documentary at home I was so

proud of him and all the family. It felt uplifting to hear people say that they had never understood MND before then and that they'd learned lessons from Rob which they could apply to their own lives. We were also boosted when Dr Jung and her colleagues told us that they had never heard MND being discussed in such detail by ordinary people.

Dr Jung was being called by people who wanted to know more about 'Rob Burrow's disease'. She smiled and said: 'Rob, you've done something that neither me nor any of my colleagues have managed after years of trying. You've shown people the reality of this disease. You have made MND famous.'

I didn't like seeing myself on screen but I had to laugh when a stranger told me that I looked taller in person than on television. I'm not sure if that was a compliment.

Years later Barrie would joke that he couldn't switch on the telly without seeing me talking about Rob or MND. He was kidding – because Barrie is a warm and high-class prankster – but he made a powerful point. Barrie understood how circumstances had changed.

I remained, essentially, a quiet and shy person. But a fire began to crackle and burn inside me.

I learned that my story is the story of so many others.

Almost five years since that first BBC documentary these shocking facts still tell a clear truth about our society and the way we live.

More than ten million people in the UK provide some kind of caring role for those they love – whether looking after family members or friends with dementia or ME, MS, MND, Parkinson's disease, cancer or heart failure – or any other of the vast array of debilitating illnesses that strike down so many of us. Perhaps these unpaid and often unrecognised people offer a few hours of support each day, or maybe they are full-time carers who attend to every single need of their loved one hour upon hour, day after day, year upon year.

The fire within me keeps burning. It is stoked by a desire to shed light on the often-forgotten role of the selfless carers who hold this country together. Without them, I know, our world would fall apart.

7

Big Hits, Babies and a Dream Home

I lay on the beautiful white sand, wearing my *Just Married* black bikini and my straw hat, barely moving. Occasionally, I would open my eyes, take off my sunglasses and turn my head to the side so that I could gaze at the turquoise sea. The longer I looked the more I saw that there were other deeper and darker shades of blue far from shore. They were so subtly different in tone that I never felt bored staring at the tranquil Indian Ocean. I didn't miss roaring and crashing waves. This was my kind of sea, as gentle as it was exquisite, and after all the excitement and stress of the wedding it was just what me and Rob needed.

We went on honeymoon to the Maldives for a week. Angsana Velavaru, which means Turtle Island in English, was a boutique-y kind of resort on a secluded island that took just five minutes to walk around. It was tiny but lovely. Everything felt perfect and discreet, from our gorgeous beach hut with the outdoor shower and cream hammock to the pristine sands, palm trees and unending sea that surrounded us. I suppose some of the real magic of the Maldives was wasted on me; I didn't want to snorkel among the colourful fish or dive along the coral reef. I was happy just basking in the sun, chatting lazily with Rob and then slipping into the water to cool off when we became too hot.

The sunsets were stunning, the evenings were cool and the food was delicious. I could not have been happier and that trip reminded us how much we loved travelling. Rob and I already knew that we wanted a family but we decided that we would pack in as many holidays as we could before life changed with the arrival of children. We loved America and in the next few years we would go to New York, Las Vegas and Florida. But we also enjoyed visiting Thailand, the Caribbean and so many countries across Europe.

Usually, we went abroad on our own but we also had some wonderful times away with friends – Angela and her boyfriend Steven, Rob's friend Jason and his wife Haley, and Natasha and Carl Ablett, who played alongside Rob for the Leeds Rhinos. Those different vacations provided the right mix of being sociable with people we liked while also making sure that some trips were just for me and Rob to have precious time together.

Rob was so busy with rugby, and his career was soaring. He was a full international and he was flying with the Rhinos as they won back-to-back Grand Finals against St Helens in 2007 and 2008. Rob won the Harry Sunderland Trophy as the Man of the Match in the first of those games, which Leeds dominated in a crushing 33–6 victory, and he was named in the Super League's Dream Team both those years. He was also Leeds' player of the season in 2007.

We still lived a very ordinary life, with Rob coming straight home after training or matches. He resisted going out with the boys, saying that he preferred being with me. We went to the movies and out for dinner, as we had become real foodies, but I didn't change much either. Rob always laughed because, even before we got to the restaurant, I would have studied the menu online and decided what I was going to order. It was all part of the anticipation for me.

When we were out and about in Castleford, Rob was often approached by fans who wandered over for a chat. They would never usually speak to someone who played for the Rhinos, their arch-enemies, but they still considered Rob a local boy. 'When are you going to come home and play for a proper team?' supporters of Castleford would ask him with broad smiles. On other occasions they would insist that they had just heard that Rob was on the verge of signing for Cas. Was it really true?

Rob laughed along with everyone, which made them even more keen that he should see the light and join Castleford. But, deep down, the Cas fans understood. The Leeds Rhinos were in the midst of building an incredible legacy. During his long career between 2004 and 2017 Rob won eight Super Leagues, three World Club Challenges and two Challenge Cups, so it was very hard for him, or any of the Rhinos, to consider life away from Leeds.

He could have accepted numerous lucrative offers from rival clubs but Rob was never going to leave the Rhinos. Like almost everyone else in the Leeds squad, he didn't even have an agent. Rob and his teammates just relied on Kevin Sinfield when they needed advice on how best to negotiate their next contract with the club. They would undoubtedly have made more money if they had brought in agents and managers but they were so united and focused as a group that those considerations mattered far less than the next trophy.

Rob and I were both happy, while remaining as quietly driven as ever. I wanted to reach new levels in physiotherapy. The plan, in another few years, was to return part-time to university while I kept working. I wanted to attain a post-grad diploma in manual therapy, which would allow me to carry the letters MACP after my name. This would grant me entry into the Musculoskeletal Association of Chartered Physiotherapists, which had around a thousand members. That's a relatively low number when you consider how many physiotherapists there are in the country and so it's an indicator of the excellence required. As well as taking various university modules, you go out on placements, where an examiner assesses the quality of your practical work in musculoskeletal physiotherapy.

My growing knowledge of spinal trauma didn't really help my anxiety when I sat in the stands at Headingley and watched Rob play. Whenever he was knocked heavily to the ground by a series of huge muscled opponents, I would wince and gasp.

Barrie McDermott remembers that Rob came to see him one day. Barrie had retired as a player but still worked with the Leeds Academy and remained a close friend and mentor to Rob.

When Rob said that he was sick of big lugs taking liberties

with him during games, Barrie shared the advice that his dad had given him. 'Find their biggest bloke,' Barrie's dad had said, 'and give him a right clump.' Barrie had said it as a joke, not expecting Rob to listen to him so closely. He could hardly believe it when soon afterwards, in a match between the Rhinos and Wigan Warriors, Rob squared up to the imposing Tongan forward Epalahame Lauaki.

It was hilarious to some as Rob, all five foot five inches of him, and weighing around ten stone six, let his punches fly after Lauaki had cuffed him round the head. Lauaki, who was half a foot taller and seven stone heavier, tried to hold him off with a meaty hand. But Rob kept fighting him and Lauaki responded with the same serious intent.

'He's coming back for more,' a commentator cackled on television while the scrap was replayed.

'I tell you what, if he had connected with that,' a co-commentator said as he admired the roundhouse right hand which Rob had just thrown amid a flurry of blows, 'Epalahame Lauaki would have been in trouble.'

His colleague kept laughing as he watched Rob fighting furiously. 'He threw so many [punches] that Lauaki thought he was surrounded. Outstanding!'

'Burrow even managed to rescue [his teammate] Keith Senior, who was struggling a little bit. Stepped in for the big fella,' the second commentator said as they revelled in the mass brawl that had broken out. Keith and many of the other Rhinos had rushed across to help Rob. But of course Rob threw more punches than anyone as he refused to be intimidated.

That bizarre scene, which showcased Rob's courage and defiance, was cherished by the Leeds faithful. But the violence of the game disturbed me. The shuddering collisions, which make rugby league so hard and unforgiving, were not entertaining online clips for me. When they involved Rob they were burned into my brain on a disturbing loop. I had witnessed the chilling sight of Rob being knocked out cold when playing for England and suffering multiple concussions for Leeds. They were distressing moments.

I went to almost every home game. All I really cared about, far more than whether the Rhinos won or lost, was that Rob walked off the pitch in one piece. Unlike me, Rob's parents Irene and Geoff had been hardcore rugby fans for years. But as the games became more brutal, I knew that, in the seat next to mine, Irene was also worried. It was terrible for her to see her son being battered and pummelled; in later years she spoke about her belief that Rob's MND might have been caused by rugby.

Nothing good can come from being tackled and hit so hard. I have also wondered about the links between rugby and the various neurological conditions that affect so many former players. We need more scientific research to know for sure, but the evidence seen by our own eyes suggests so much.

Beyond damage done to the brain I was always concerned about the state of Rob's neck, back and spine. And even when I knew that the injuries would heal, and not result in impaired cognitive powers or the threat of potential paralysis, it was still upsetting to see Rob break a bone while playing a game. I remember watching an away match on television and, after another crunching tackle, Rob took a long time to get up. He was soon surrounded by the medics and, when he finally walked slowly off the field, holding his limp arm, it was obvious that he had broken his collarbone.

Each year became harder. When he was younger Rob seemed able to spring up faster. There was far less medical care then – after a bang to the head, they would wave some smelling salts under his nose and he'd plunge back into the game without passing any concussion protocols.

My anxiety drained the enjoyment out of watching Rob playing rugby. I would spend most of the match yearning for the final whistle. Rob understood my concerns and, soon after he stepped off the pitch, he followed the same ritual. He would walk straight across to his bag in the dressing room and reach for his phone. Within a few minutes of the game ending, my mobile would ping with a text from Rob assuring me that he was fine.

These are some of the hidden doubts and fears that people don't often think about, let alone see, when they consider the 'dream life' of playing, and earning a good living in, professional sport. It's the same when people look back fondly at a great sporting career once it's over. Rob won so much with the Rhinos that many of the fans remain unaware of his pain and frustration when he was used so often as a substitute from the bench.

Rob was usually so good in being able to keep his rugby career and our home lives in completely separate compartments. Whenever he got home to Pontefract he left his rugby headaches in Leeds. But it eventually became impossible to hide how much the situation at work was affecting him and it was important that I offered the support and understanding he often needed during these more challenging periods of his career.

There was disappointment too in some international matches. Despite having been Leeds' player of the season, Rob wasn't picked to play in any of England's games while on a tour of Australia and New Zealand. Brian Noble, the head coach, chose not to select him and Rob was devastated. He confided in Jamie Peacock, his Leeds teammate and one of the sport's great players, who also couldn't fathom why Rob was being ignored.

In later years, Noble said that whenever he went through footage of his squad in training or the dressing room on that tour, he was struck by the fact that Rob was such a positive and lively presence. He was always making everyone laugh, while delighting in their successes, because he refused to sulk about his personal disappointment.

That reaction summed up Rob's character and explained why I was so proud of him. It was harder for him at Leeds because once Brian McDermott became head coach of the Rhinos in 2011, Rob's position became muddled. He was part of such an impressive squad and it was unfortunate that three brilliant players – Kev Sinfield, Danny McGuire and Rob – were sometimes competing for two places in the starting thirteen. Rob was the Rhinos number 7 for most of his career, with his number suggesting that he was still regarded as the starting scrum half. But Brian didn't see it that way.

Rob's most memorable match was certainly the 2011 Grand

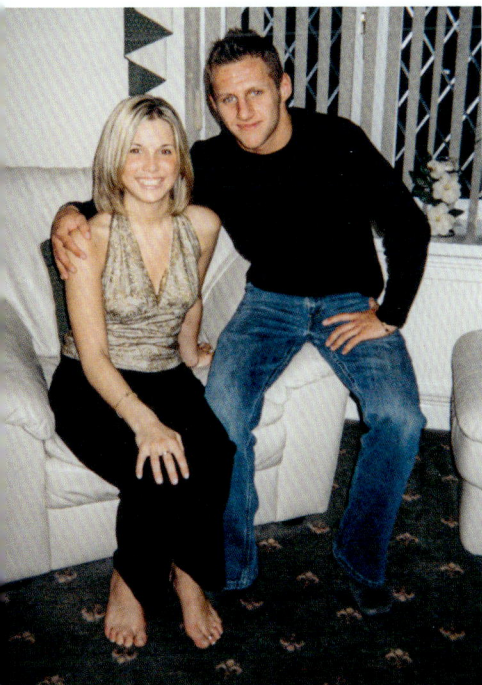

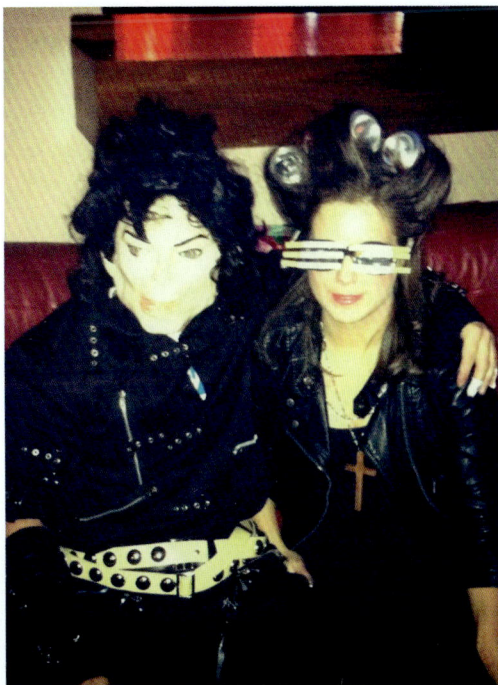

oung love. I had first gone out with Rob
hen we were fifteen. We ended up living
ogether for more than half of our adult
ves. There are so many snapshots of joy in
y head.

We loved fancy dress. Rob, of course, dressed
up here as his pop icon, Michael Jackson.
Me: cans for hair rollers and cigarettes on my
sunglasses. What was I thinking? Maybe Lady
Gaga approves.

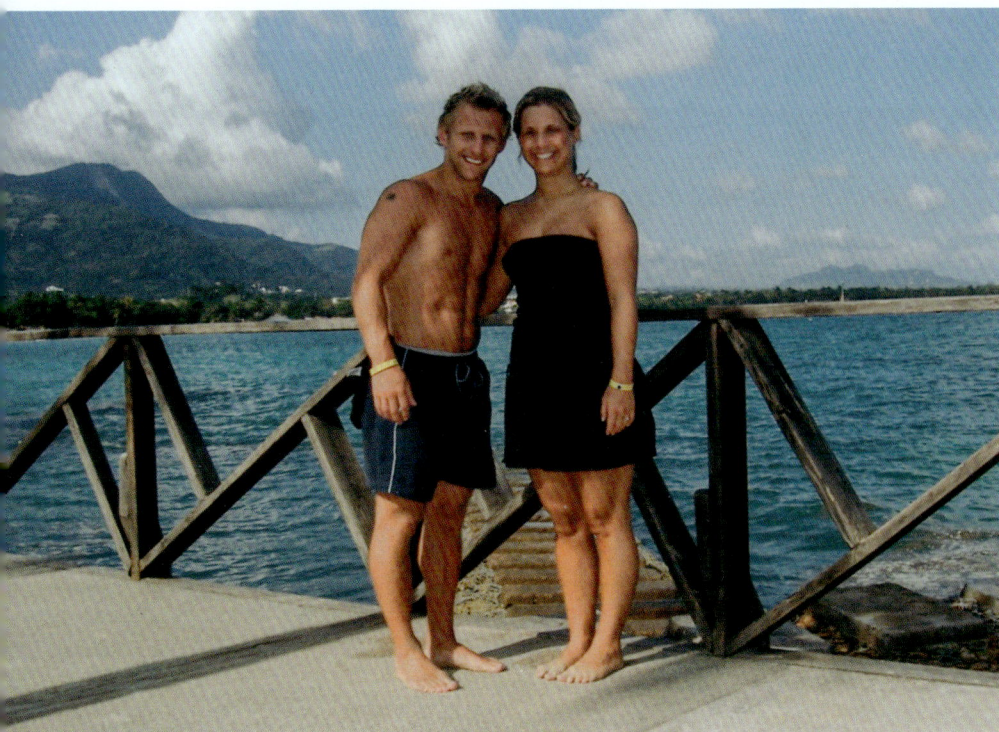

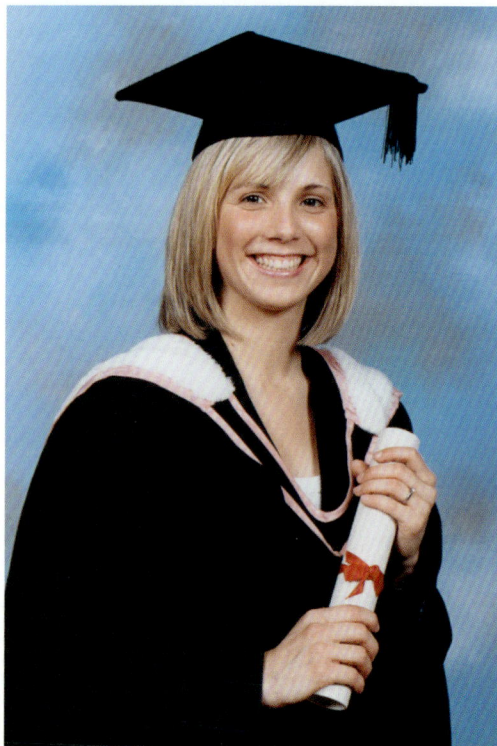

July 2004: Manchester University, graduation day. This was such a proud moment for me on my way to qualifying as a physiotherapist.

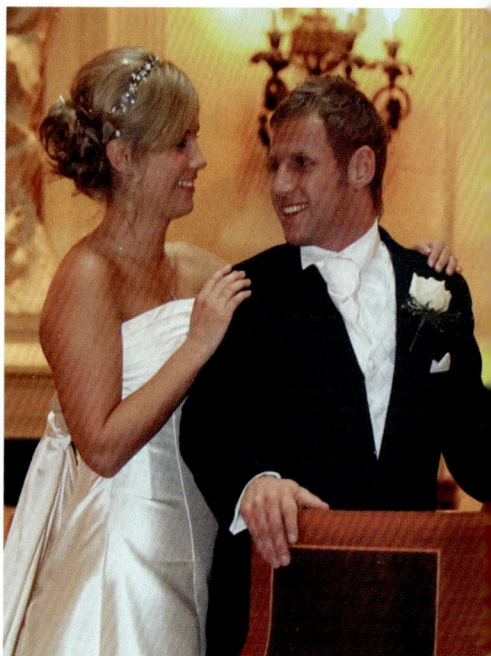

30 December 2006: St John the Evangelist Church, Leeds. There was something so romantic about getting married on a cold but beautifully sunlit afternoon in Yorkshire. I know every couple say this, but it *really* was one of the happiest days of our lives.

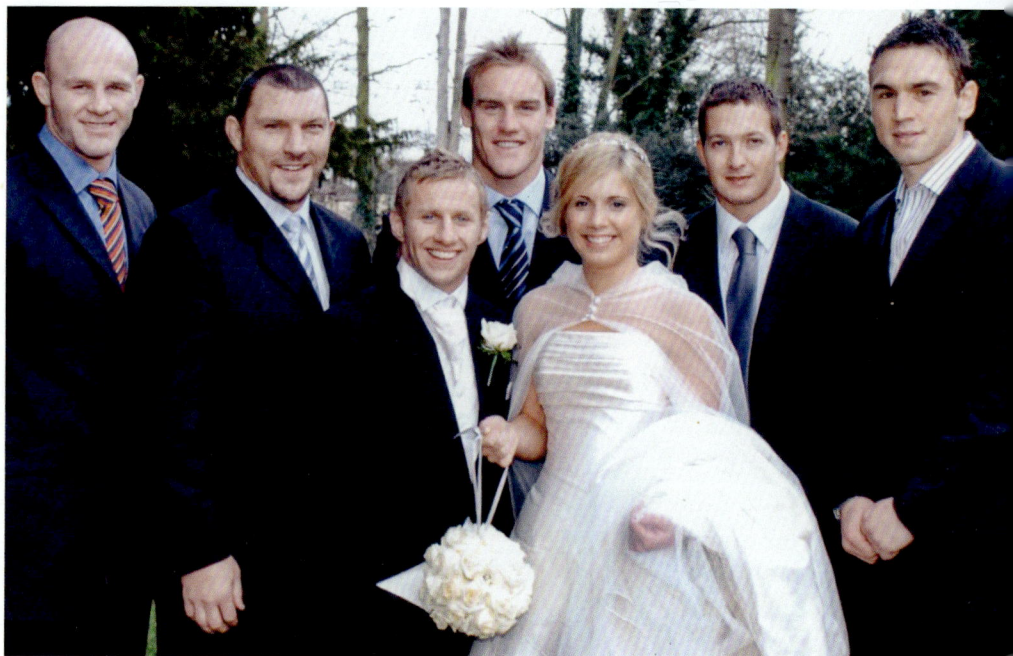

Rob and I with his Leeds Rhinos teammates, from left to right: Keith Senior, Barrie McDermott, Gareth Ellis, Danny McGuire and Kevin Sinfield.

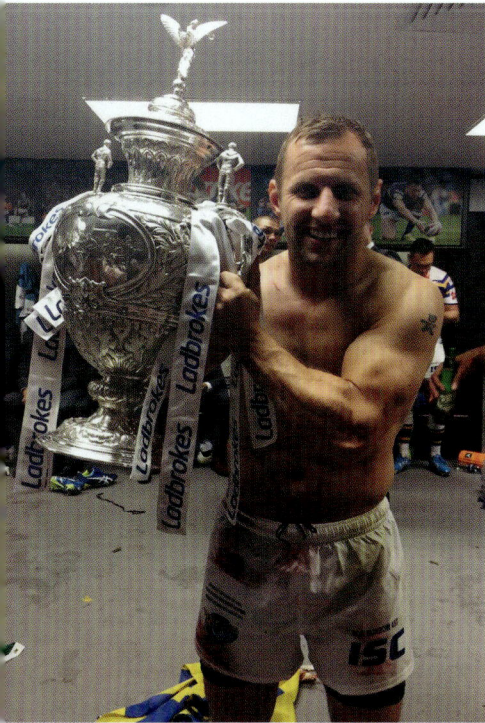

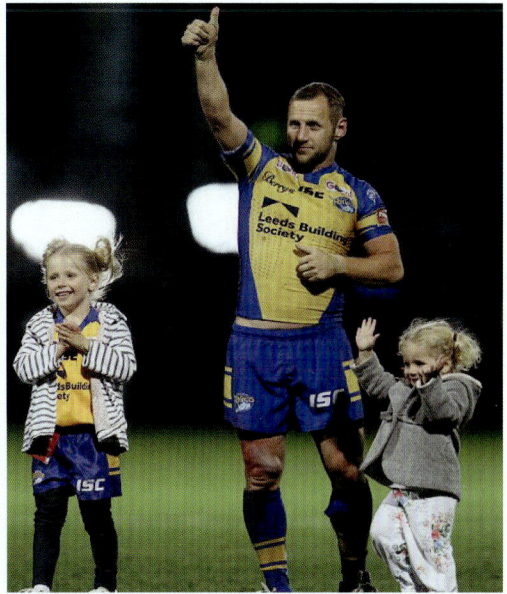

After his family and me, the Leeds Rhinos were the love of Rob's life. He joined their Academy in 1999 and spent the next eighteen years, and his entire professional career, at Leeds.

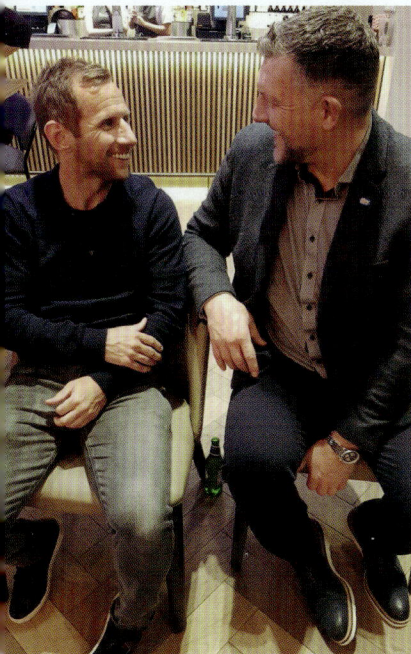

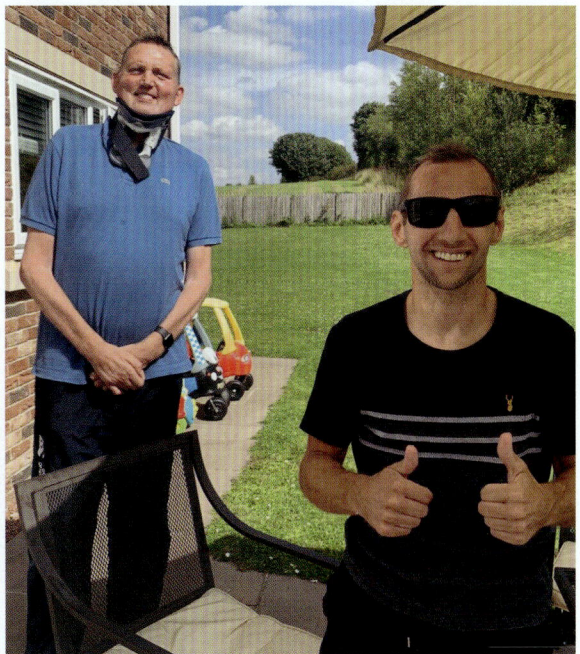

(*Left*) Rob with former teammate and friend Barrie McDermott. (*Right*) Rob with Doddie Weir, another rugby legend and brilliant ambassador for the MND community. Rob valued Doddie's friendly good cheer and openness with his own experiences of living with the disease. They knew little about each other's code of rugby – beyond that they were physical and brutal games. Doddie reminded Rob that they had both taken some almighty hits and been knocked to the ground, but still they'd got up. They'd fought on.

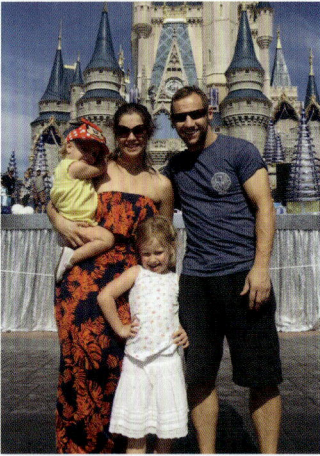

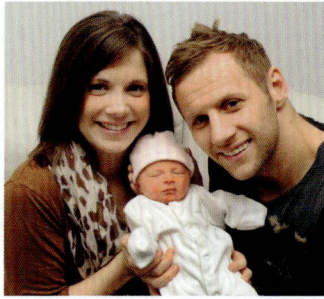

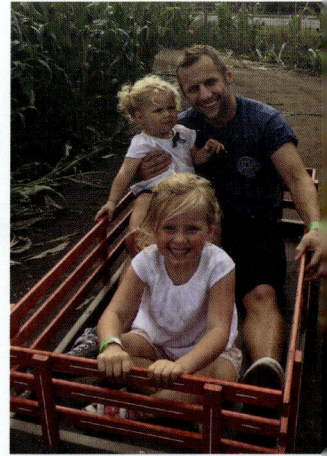

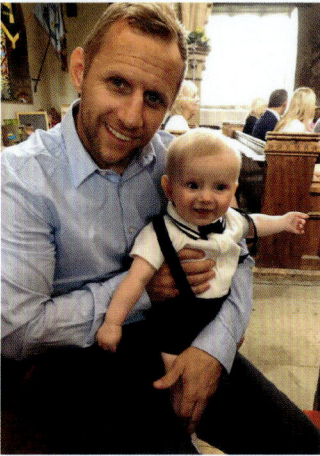

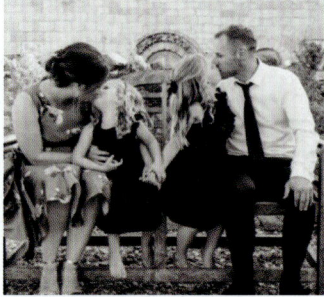

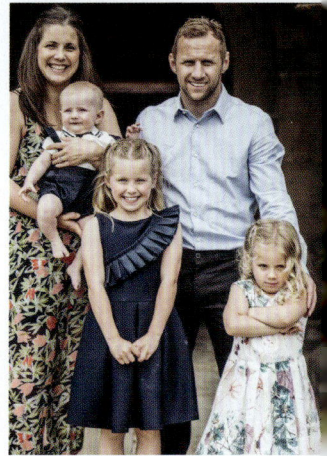

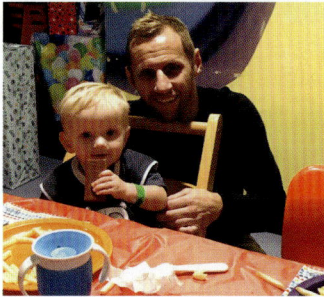

Rob and I became the parents of three beautiful children: Macy, Maya and Jackson. Family was everything to Rob and his character shines through them. Our children were fortunate to have a mum and a dad who were around so much, and we have some wonderful memories together.

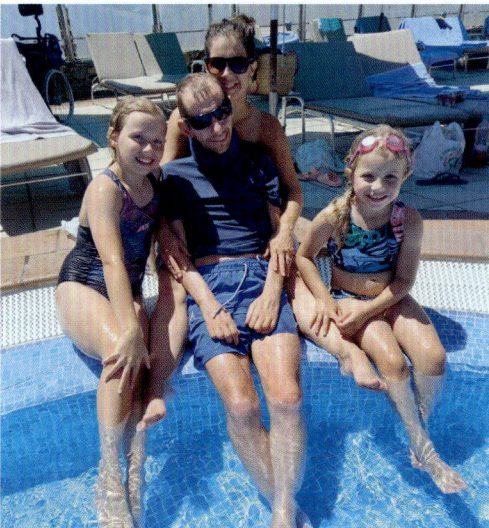

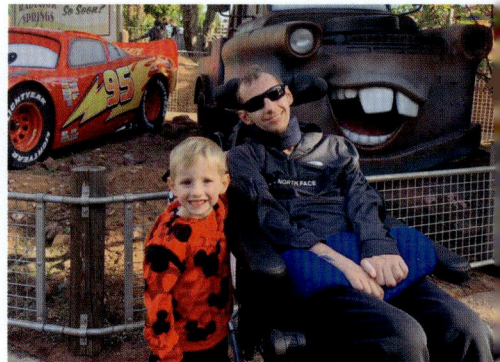

We bought a villa close to Disney World in Florida, where we shared many holidays as a family, including after Rob's diagnosis. It's a magical place for us. Rob proposed to me there, all those years ago!

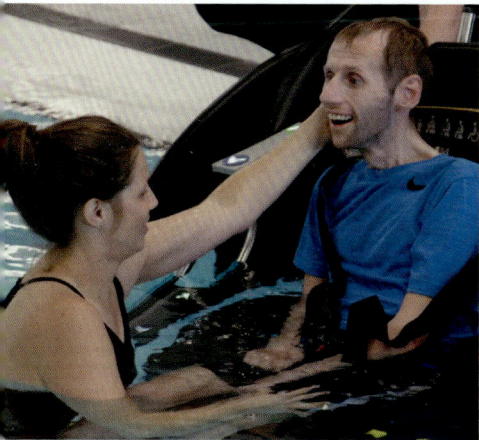
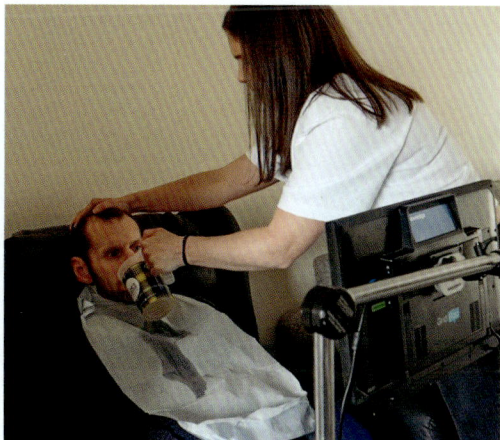

ob made me feel so lucky to have loved him for twenty-six years and to be in a position where could care for him.

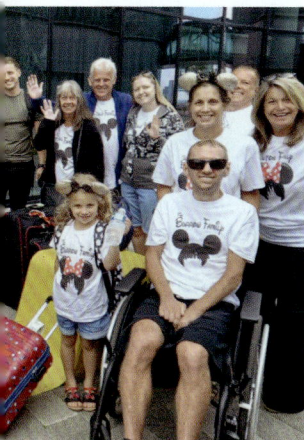
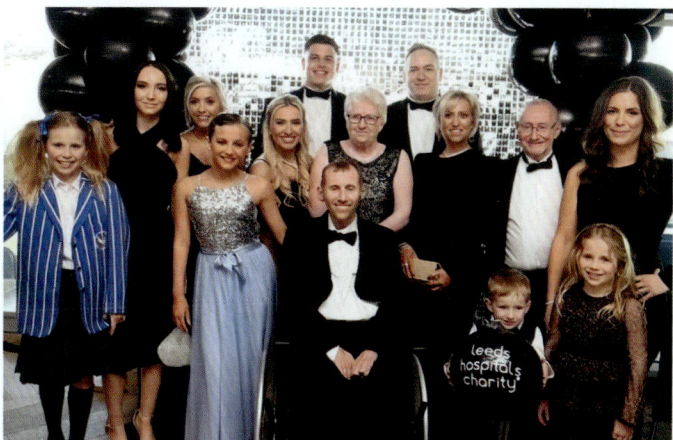

ine and Rob's families have been a rock of support. I will always be grateful for their love and e help that they continue to give to me and the children.

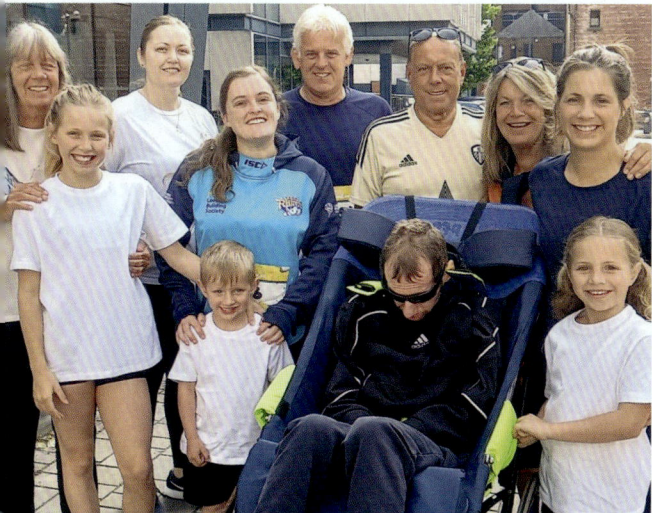
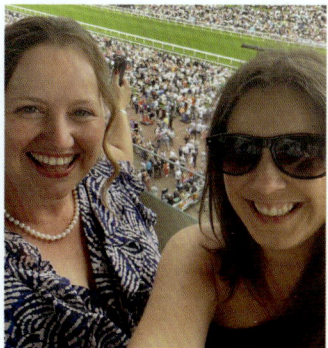

Enjoying a day at the races with my best friend, Angela. She has been there through the good times and bad – a friend like this is hard to find.

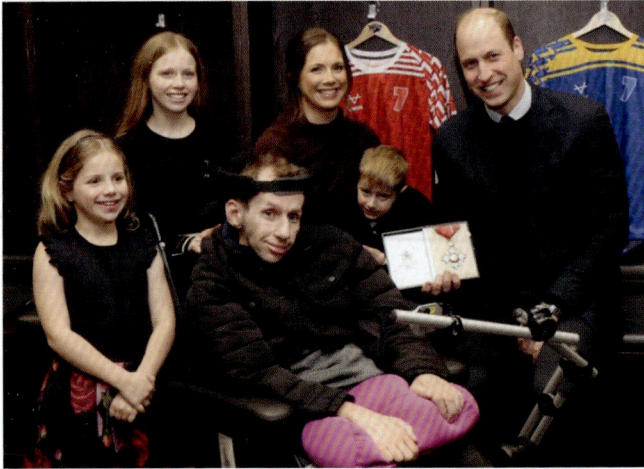

It was a special moment when HRH Prince William awarded Rob and Kev their CBEs at Headingley Stadium. This is a treasured family photo from that day. The children were so excited to come along!

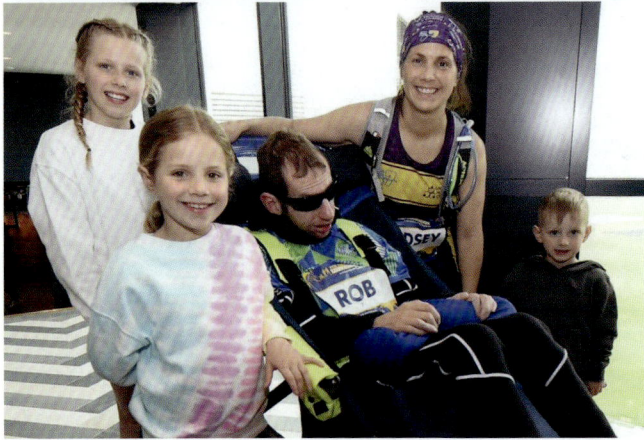

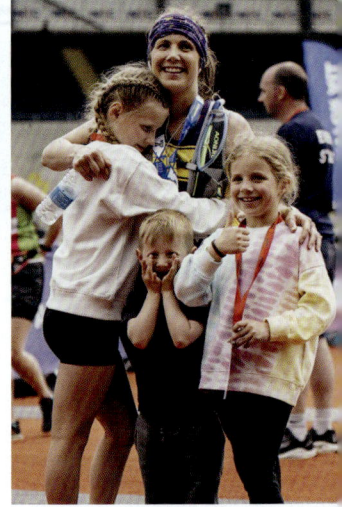

Taking part in the 2023 Rob Burrow Leeds Marathon was a great challenge. My heartfelt thank you to all those who have supported Rob, Kev and I in our fundraising journey for MND. I know it meant a lot to Rob too; I'm so proud of how he became such an inspiring ambassador for the MND community.

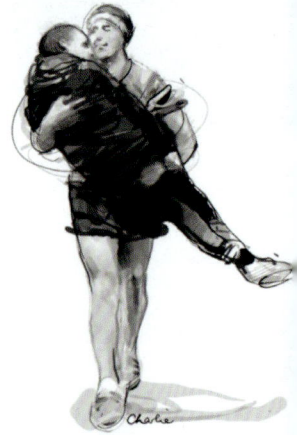

Kevin Sinfield and Rob Burrow

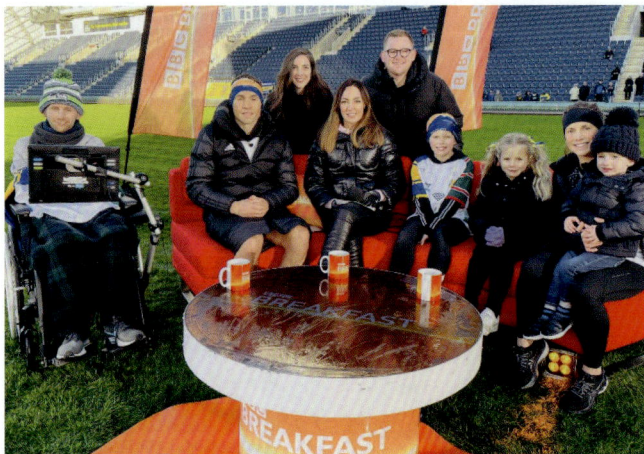

at The Rob Burrow Leeds Marathon ♡

Kev and Rob finishing the Leeds Marathon together over the line. Beautifully illustrated by the artist Charlie Mackesy.

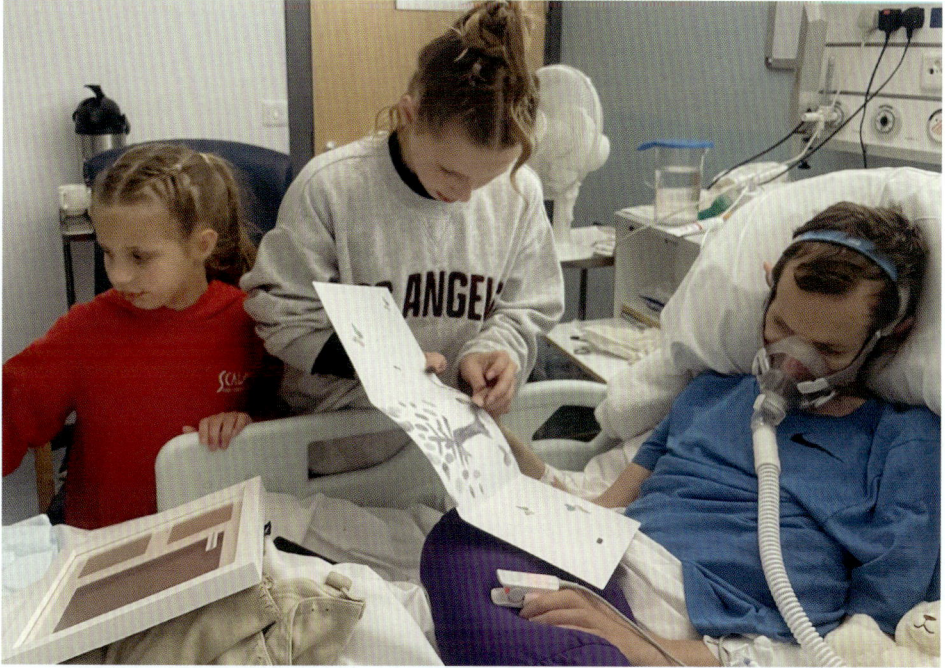

1 July 2024: Pinderfields Hospital, Wakefield. Rob's last night with the family. The nurses had brought the children ink pads, which you normally use to make prints of a newborn baby's tiny hands and feet. Macy made a little tree out of his fingerprints. Rob was awake but drowsy as he watched the children having fun and making prints for their memory books. The nurses had also given the children tiny knitted hearts and bears to take home. I took so many photos of Rob and the children together. In the last photograph I ever took of Rob he is smiling, surrounded by love and his three children.

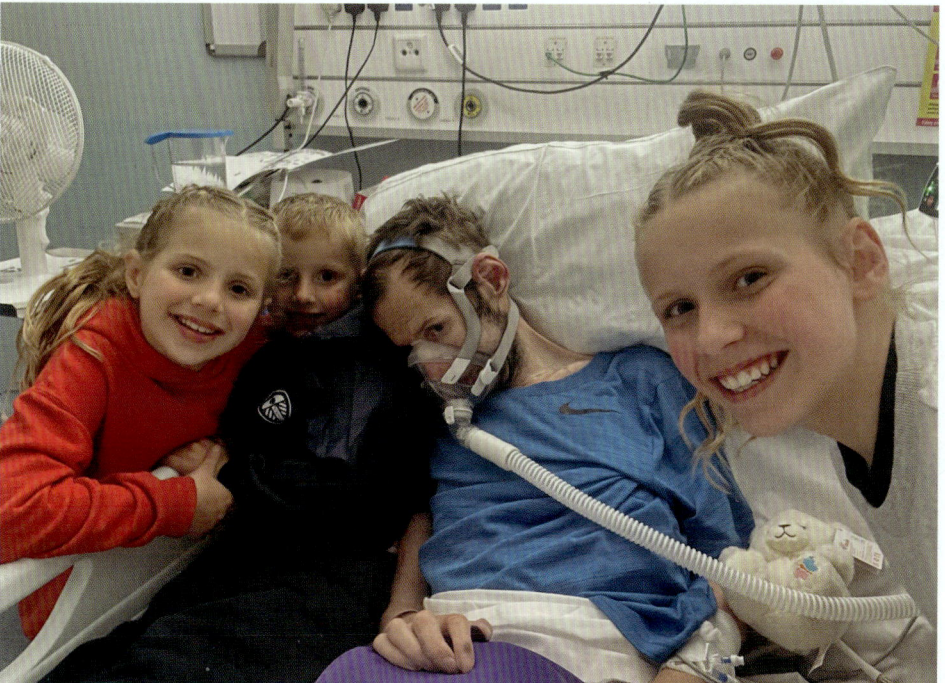

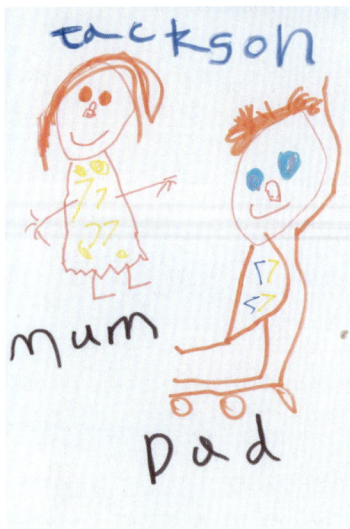

A drawing of Mum and Dad by Jackson, aged 5.

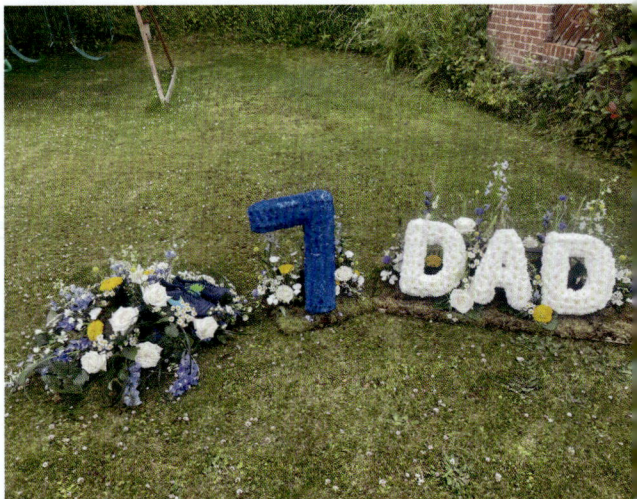

The flowers in the garden before we left for Rob's funeral, together with his first ever rugby boots, the last pair he ever wore and his shirt number 7 from the Rhinos.

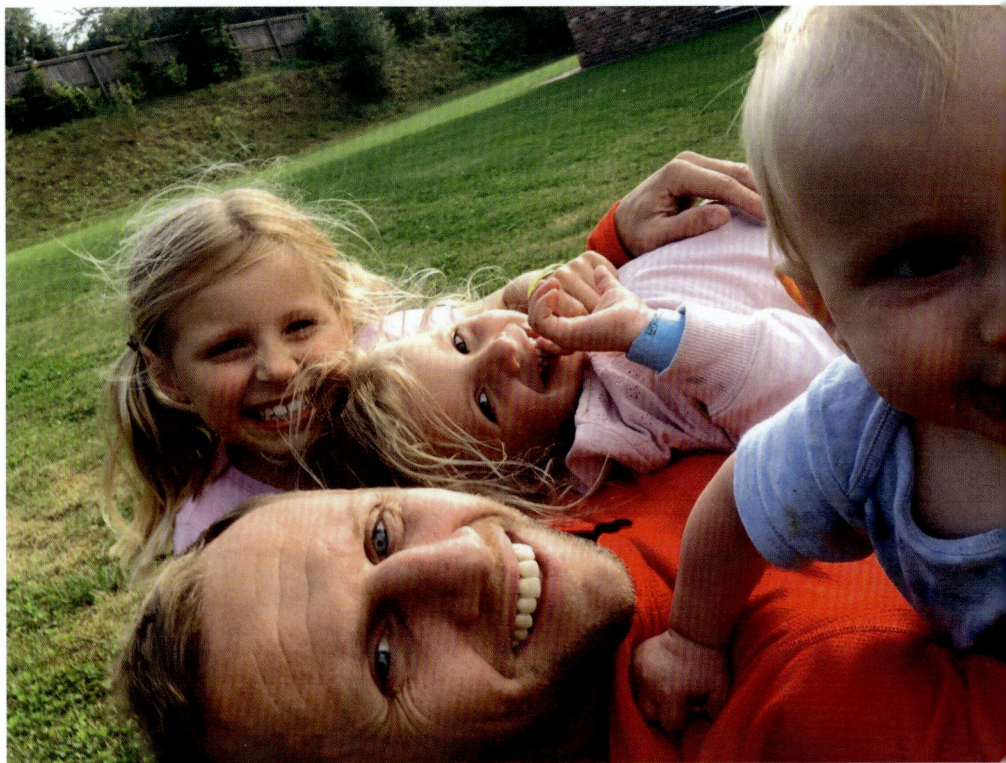

Some of Macy and Maya's beautiful words at the funeral for Rob:

Thank you for being our dad and for looking after us. You are without doubt the most bravest, loved dad in the whole world. I hope I grow up to be just like you.

We love you, Dad, and we miss you, but we know that you will be with us every step of the way.

Daddy, you will continue to inspire us every day and we will do our best to always make you prou…

Final, when he came on to inspire Leeds against St Helens. Barrie McDermott (who, though he shared the name of the new coach, was no relation) sat high up in the commentary box for Sky Sports at Old Trafford. It was a struggle for him not to leap out of his chair and scream with joy when Rob set off on that blistering and jinking run through the Saints defence to score what is now routinely described as the greatest Grand Final try in history. Barrie had to simply clench his fist in triumph beneath the table as most of the 70,000 fans, besides the Saints supporters, went crazy. Rob then set up another try for Leeds as they came back and romped home 32–16.

Faye Peacock, Jamie's wife, turned to me late on in the game to say that Rob had just won his second Harry Sunderland Trophy as Man of the Match in a Grand Final. My knowledge of rugby remained sketchy, but even I could tell that Faye was right. I felt ecstatic for Rob and, in a rare break from worrying about him being hurt, I could enjoy the rest of the game.

Afterwards Rob was his usual modest self as he tried to downplay the significance of his performance. But I think Barrie was right when he said Rob played with a real sense of anger that day. He always stood up for himself and he had challenged Brian repeatedly about not starting matches. Brian was a tough man, a former marine and rugby league player who'd had his share of battles with Barrie when they'd faced each other in the past, and he was not about to back down. So when Rob took to the field in the first half he was determined to play with fire and purpose and try to convince Brian that he should start every game from then on.

He produced a performance for the ages. Rob also fulfilled the prediction that Danny McGuire had made the night before. They had shared a room and Danny tried to boost his friend's morale when he promised Rob that he would come on and win the game for Leeds.

Barrie empathised with Rob whenever he was consigned to the bench. But he knew that his little pal was all right when he heard the stories that confirmed that Rob remained the chief prankster and indestructible joker at the heart of the Rhinos dressing room.

Kylie Leuluai, the formidable New Zealand prop, joined Leeds in 2007 and played alongside Rob for the next eight years. He was the biggest Rhino of them all and he took Barrie's place in bearing the brunt of Rob's wisecracks. Kylie was run ragged but he still loved Rob. Their most infamous comic spat occurred on a day when Rob had teased Kylie mercilessly in training. Kylie put him in a chokehold as a little reminder that enough was enough.

Rob would not allow Kylie to have the upper hand for long and so he banked the chokehold in his memory and began plotting a devilish act of revenge. It required great patience and ingenuity over the next few days.

Using a heavy-duty hole punch, he went to work on hundreds of sheets of white paper. Page after page was punched countless times. Rob gathered thousands of little circles of white paper, which he then hid in the air vents of Kylie's car.

An hour later a cheerful and oblivious Kylie climbed into his car, turned on the ignition and was immediately covered in a blizzard of paper. When Kylie stumbled out of the car, confused and stunned by the mysterious attack, Rob was in hysterics. It looked as if Kylie had been hit by a tsunami of confetti at a particularly drunken wedding.

Rob delighted in the precision of his planning and execution. But his helpless laughter soon had Kylie roaring and chasing after him again.

Rob and I became more serious as we decided to start a family in 2011. We had been married for four and a half years and were both about to turn twenty-nine. After all the holidays and good times we wanted to share our happiness with two or three children. I fell pregnant quickly, within a month of trying to conceive, and we were very excited. We only shared the news with our parents and siblings and everyone was thrilled.

I felt well and we agreed that I would keep working as long as possible before giving birth. We had everything mapped out and the first ten weeks of my pregnancy felt like a breeze. I had my twelve-week scan booked in and I had started to feel a tingle as I imagined the tiny baby growing inside me. I dreamed of how I might look when I started to show off a little bump.

My mum and I went to a concert together and all felt good until I reached the toilet at the venue. I noticed that I had started spotting and a shiver of trepidation ran through me. But I reminded myself to stay calm, go home and get some rest. As long as I took it easy and didn't do anything silly, I was sure everything would be fine.

It was good to be back home with Rob and he made sure

that I put my feet up and relaxed before we went to bed. I still felt okay and fell asleep soon after we switched off the lights.

But then, everything changed. I woke up in the dead of night. The pain was of such intensity that I now think that it was worse than childbirth itself. I spent a long time in the bathroom, Rob trying to comfort me while I was hunched over in agony. I knew the baby and I were in trouble but I could barely speak. The pain became raw and crippling.

I remember crying on the bathroom floor as I began to haemorrhage. There was so much blood and I knew what it meant. We had lost the baby.

Rob looked helpless and bereft. 'Get my mum and dad,' I managed to say.

I lay on the floor, the pool of blood spreading around me, as I heard Rob's urgent conversation with my mum.

My parents arrived fifteen minutes later; by then, Rob had carried me to bed and wiped away most of the blood. I curled up in bed, looking ashen and anguished, while my mum and dad tried to comfort me. They said that it was important that I went to hospital. The baby was gone but I needed to be looked after.

Rob drove me to Pinderfields, the new hospital in Wakefield, with my parents following. The roads looked ghostly and deserted at three in the morning. We didn't say much in the car but Rob kept glancing at me. Sometimes he'd ask if I was okay or just stretch out his hand to me. The street lights cast eerie shadows across our faces but, while I was full of deep sadness, I also felt the love between us. Rob's care and support helped and I wanted to tell him not to worry. We would get through this and have a baby one day. But I felt too weak to talk. I just squeezed his hand back and tried to deal with the spasms of pain that still rippled through me.

At Pinderfields the nurses and doctors were extraordinarily kind and attentive. My mum remembers that as they had run out of note paper, one of the nurses wrote down all my details on a blue paper towel. I was too distressed to even notice. But I soon began to calm myself as they confirmed I would not need a D&C, which is a minor surgical procedure.

I couldn't help myself. I blurted out the question that already consumed me: 'When can I try for another baby?'

My mum was surprised and expected that I would be told to remain patient. She was sure that they would recommend me waiting for at least six months.

But the hospital bolstered me. They said I was fit and well and that as soon as I recovered from the miscarriage, there were no physical reasons that would delay our trying again.

I felt a great weight lift from me. Amid the lingering hurt, there was hope too.

Rob and I would still become parents. The hope turned into conviction and that inner certainty helped me accept the loss, and that, in turn, lifted Rob's spirits. We were going to be all right.

The hospital staff were soon proved right. A few months later we learned that I was pregnant again. There was a little anxiety, which was natural after all we had been through, but we decided to press ahead with the short break we had booked even before the miscarriage. A P&O cruise would take us from Hull to Bruges in Belgium when I was around ten weeks into my second pregnancy. I convinced Rob that we should go.

A few days before the cruise I noticed small signs of spotting. I was terrified and called Rob. He immediately drove across to pick me up from work at the Chapel Allerton Hospital in Leeds and made me feel much better. I was due my first twelve-week NHS scan soon after we returned from Bruges but Rob insisted that we take no chances. We booked me in for a private scan the following evening.

It was very hard waiting almost a full day for the scan. But as soon as we saw images of the baby, and were told by the smiling sonographer that everything looked great, relief flooded through us. We could feel excited again about having a baby.

The rest of my pregnancy was trouble-free – apart from the fact that I had terrible eczema on my face. It was so itchy that I couldn't stop scratching. I remember being in Paris with Rob and we walked past a garage, which had one side covered in a giant mirror. I caught sight of my reflection and was shocked by how horrible I looked. Rob tried to tell me that I was still beautiful but I sobbed my heart out. It looked like my face had been rubbed raw with sandpaper.

I was in the middle of doing my MSc and was on clinical placement too. Perhaps the stress of working so hard, while being back at uni part-time and doing my exams, caused the eczema. Or maybe it was just a consequence of all the hormones raging through me. I just knew I looked horrendous; when I look back at photographs of that time, I can see that I was not just being emotional during my pregnancy. My eczema really had been very bad.

Three weeks before my due date, the wives and girlfriends of the Leeds players had arranged a baby shower for me at Banyan, a bar and restaurant located in a stately old post office in Roundhay. It was a lovely setting and I was looking forward to seeing everyone. But that morning, my waters broke. Rob rushed me to hospital but the midwife was relaxed and thought it would be another twenty-four hours before I gave birth. She advised me to go home and get on with the rest of my day.

Once we were home I called my mum. She was shocked that I was still planning to go to the baby shower. I pointed out that, as this was my first baby, the hospital were confident that I would not be in full-blown labour for another day. I could make it to the baby shower as planned.

'But, Lindsey, you don't want to risk infection,' my mum warned.

'Oh, Mum, I'm fine,' I said. 'I'm still going tonight.'

Mum hung up and, when they heard the news, her colleagues at the school kept saying: 'Your Lindsey can't be doing that.'

But there was no one, apart from Rob, who knew me as well as my mum. She could tell that my mind was made up and so she and Dad came over that evening. Along with Rob, they would accompany me to the baby shower, which showed how worried they were about me. They were relieved, at least, that Rob was not leaving for Cyprus in the morning. He had been due to travel to a training camp but Brian McDermott agreed that he was needed more at home. If my waters had broken a couple of days later Rob would have been in Cyprus – we got lucky.

I had twinges all through the baby shower but there was nothing too dramatic and everyone made a fuss of me. We left a little earlier than planned as the pain began to bite. On the journey home it was tough not to cry out with every bump in the road.

As soon as we made it home I went straight to bed while my parents drove back to Castleford to wait for news. In the early hours of the morning I could stand it no longer.

'We have to go now, Rob,' I urged.

Rob helped me into the car and we raced through the dark to hospital. It was not easy when the midwife examined me and said I still had a little way to go.

I think Rob found it almost as hard as I did. He kept asking me to have something for the pain. I was so adamant about the kind of natural birth I wanted that I hissed at him: 'Rob, if you mention pain relief once more, I swear that I won't take it, whatever happens tonight.'

Rob knew how stubborn I could be and so he was much quieter from then on. He just allowed me to squeeze his hand really hard while I tried to control my breathing and the pain.

The next few hours were a blur. But I can remember vividly now the cries of delight, replacing my muffled howl, when our baby arrived after a straightforward birth. Most of all I remember the look of wonder and love on Rob's face as he stared at our little girl and then at me.

'You did it, Lindsey,' he said as he hugged and kissed me, laughing and crying at the same time. 'She's here. And she's just as beautiful as you.'

Life at home with Rob and Macy was a joy, as we entered a new stage of our lives. We had become a family and the years stretched out in front of us with glorious promise. Rob and I wanted two more children as five of us would make a great little team. He threw himself into fatherhood and tried to be at home as much as he could to push the pram, play with Macy, help change her nappies and feed her, all while making sure that I was doing well as a new mum.

It also helped that Rob was starting regularly for the Rhinos and making a significant contribution every week – even though it had caused much unhappiness when Brian McDermott moved him to hooker. Rob saw himself as a pure scrum half playing alongside his old mate Danny McGuire at stand-off, which is a key position where the tactician of the team makes crucial decisions in how best to launch attacks.

But when Rob looked at the changed team sheet his name was usually between two props in Kylie and Jamie Peacock. Kev had moved from loose forward to stand-off and he played in tandem with Danny, who was switched to scrum half. The Rhinos remained a formidable team.

With Rob starting as a hooker, while still wearing his old number 7 shirt, Leeds had another outstanding season in 2012. They won the World Club Challenge in February when they beat Manly, the Australian champions, at Headingley. Eight months later they brought the season to a familiar thrilling climax as they won yet another Grand Final after beating Warrington Wolves. Rob was on from the start as hooker and Kev won the Harry Sunderland Trophy with a mighty performance, despite taking some heavy hits in the game.

These were the golden years of the long and extraordinary reign of the Rhinos. But I still worried about Rob because he was never made to feel secure in his position by Brian McDermott. Uncertainty always seemed to stalk him, no matter how well he played, and Rob could never be sure that his coach truly backed him.

But there could be little arguing about their sustained success. The Rhinos were supreme in Super League. They had won five of the last six Grand Finals, and six of the previous nine.

Yet even giants can be fallible. The Challenge Cup was the trophy they found hardest to win – Leeds played five finals between 2000 and 2013 and lost them all. It was strange: even if it did not match the season-long grind of becoming Super League champions in the Grand Final, the Challenge Cup was a landmark on the rugby calendar every year.

In August 2014, at Wembley, Rob started in the final as hooker against my childhood team, Castleford Tigers. The Challenge Cup hoodoo hung over the Rhinos, but a team packed with men of such resolve and talent were not about to surrender again to the rugby gods. They won the competition for the first time in fifteen years, sealing a comfortable victory when Danny, having cracked three ribs earlier in the game, slotted a drop goal in the seventy-seventh minute. We could all finally relax and celebrate as little Macy danced a jig on my lap.

Rob, Danny, Kev, Jamie Jones-Buchanan and Ryan Bailey had played in all six of those previous defeats and so relief after breaking that long losing streak poured out of them. 'You dream of being able to enjoy the last few minutes,' Kev said on television after the game. 'I'd describe this as a reward for perseverance, not just of the players but the coaching staff and the fans who've spent their hard-earned cash driving down the M1 so many times and gone back disillusioned. Hopefully they're happy tonight.'

We were thrilled and, a year later, the Rhinos won their second straight Challenge Cup as they stampeded over Hull Kingston Rovers and won 50–0. It was just a touch disappointing for us as Rob was on the bench at the start – but he came on and scored a sparkling late try.

The Rhinos ended that season on an almost impossible high when the Grand Final against Wigan provided an unforgettable send-off for Kev, Kylie and Jamie Peacock. Kev, at thirty-five, was two years older than Rob, while the old warriors Kylie and Jamie were both thirty-seven. In a clear sign that an era was closing at Leeds, Kev was about to switch codes and play rugby union for the Rhinos' sister club Yorkshire Carnegie. Jamie was preparing to become a coach at Hull KR, while Kylie had decided to retire from the game entirely.

Rob started at hooker and an epic final unfolded. Leeds were 16–6 up at half-time but then all their efforts over such a long and successful season appeared to catch up with them. The

Rhinos began to flag and, within eight minutes of the second half, Wigan surged into a four-point lead. It looked as if the Warriors had built an unstoppable momentum but the grit of the Rhinos was remarkable. They dug in, stemmed the tide, and then produced some blue-and-amber magic as Josh Walters scored the winning try in a 22–20 victory.

Leeds had just won the treble, becoming only the third side in history to win the Challenge Cup, the League Leaders Shield (awarded to the team finishing top of the league at the end of the regular season) and the Grand Final in the same year. 'Without a doubt it's the perfect ending,' Kev said just before he lifted the trophy in front of 74,000 people at Old Trafford. 'To top it off with the treble in the final year is unbelievable, and I'm so thankful I've been able to play alongside this group every single week. These memories stay with you for ever, and it's something I'll cherish for ever.'

Danny McGuire, who won the Harry Sunderland Trophy, suggested that they were the best team in the history of the club: 'Achievements like today leave us right at the top. There's three of my best mates leaving this club and I just wanted to play as well as I could and run my blood to water for this team. They deserved to go out on a high.'

The loss of three key players knocked the Rhinos off course. Leeds struggled in 2016 and finished fourth bottom in the table. They lost fifteen out of their twenty-three Super League games and Rob, who was so used to playing in a dominant team, found it difficult. He still managed to shield the family from his work problems but there were times when I could tell he was preoccupied.

Rob played twenty-eight games for Leeds across all competitions and started in all but one that year. He scored six tries but he knew the end of his career was looming too, and he sometimes felt as if his body was in pieces. I could see how much he suffered.

When Maya was born she brought even more delight into our personal lives. Family life was blissful but the pain of rugby could not be escaped, as hard as Rob tried to hide it. He wanted to be active with the girls and run around with four-year-old Macy but it was becoming increasingly difficult. It took him longer to recover from a game and I could see the physical effects, which reminded me of the claim that playing a full-blown game of professional rugby has the equivalent impact of your body going through multiple car crashes over the course of eighty minutes.

A G-force of forty is usually felt during a car accident at forty miles per hour – and, for passengers wearing a seatbelt, blunt force trauma occurs when the speed of the vehicle is at fifty miles per hour. Serious injuries and fatalities occur when the G-force hits seventy. Apparently – and I've obviously never seen proof of this myself – the highest-ever G-force recorded on a rugby field is 205.

I could see how difficult it was for Rob to get out of bed the morning after a game. He had signed his Academy contract at the age of twelve and made his first team debut in 2001 when he was nineteen. At the end of the 2016 season he was thirty-four and knew he had just one more year as a player left in him. Rob had been through hundreds of car-crash collisions with opponents – most of whom weighed six or seven stone more than him – and too many concussive incidents.

He began 2017 with a determination to make it a season to remember. Despite Rob's continued excellence for the Rhinos, he had become a 'finisher', as substitutes are now called, rather than a guaranteed starter. He played twenty-four games and only started ten. Rob still scored nine tries, and kicked five goals, to contribute forty-six points.

He also always looked for me and the girls in the crowd so that he could give us a special wave. And whenever he took another big hit he made sure to give me a reassuring nod, once back on his feet.

Rob's starting situation actually worsened because his speed and trickery were used to cut a tiring opposition defence to shreds. As his rivals flagged there was often no stopping Rob: feeling fresh and out to prove a point, he would come on and often win the game for Leeds. In a strange way that seemed to work against him because Brian could argue that the strategy was clearly working.

Rob was in a no-win situation and he regularly spoke to me and Barrie about his frustration. He was becoming increasingly disillusioned because he sensed that Brian was playing mind games with him. Rob felt it was unfair and, while I'm obviously biased, I don't think Brian handled the situation well, but it was obviously not my place to say anything to anyone at the club. I also understood that, as a coach at elite level, Brian had to make difficult selection choices every week. But, after all his years at Leeds, Rob deserved better treatment. At the very least he deserved clear but supportive communication.

I would get angry because I saw Rob's love for the game dwindling. It also upset me because Rob never gave less than 100 per cent and he poured everything of himself into the club. But Brian's attitude was having a marked effect on Rob.

I believe that Rob's decision to retire was prompted by the difficulties he endured under Brian. For the first time in his career he wondered if playing on was worth the hurt; ultimately, he decided he'd had enough of it all.

His old friend understood because, at the end of his own career, Barrie was also often benched at a time when Brian was the assistant to Tony Smith, the Australian coach. Barrie respected Tony but that did not make his disappointment any easier to bear when, in his final season for Leeds, he was left out of the squad for the final of the 2005 Challenge Cup. Rob started at scrum half that day while Barrie had been mortified when he'd received the news of his exclusion. His whole family had travelled to Cardiff for the final at the Millennium Stadium and so Barrie confided in Rob. It was the one occasion where their usual roles were swapped as Rob counselled and consoled Barrie.

Leeds suffered heartbreak in the end, too, as they lost the Cup to Hull by a single point, 25–24.

Barrie reminded Rob of those moments as a way of saying that the pain would pass. He just needed to give the very best of himself, control his own preparations and performances and not worry too much about the rest of it. He would find a way. Rob processed everything and, as he could be rational and pragmatic rather than just a cheeky little mischief-maker, he had already reached the same conclusion.

It helped that Leeds hauled themselves back into contention once more in 2017. There were some bad days – with the worst being their 66–10 loss away to Castleford in March – but Rob, Danny, Jamie Jones-Buchanan, Carl Ablett, Ryan Hall, Tom Briscoe and the other leading Rhinos refused to give in. The Rhinos finished second at the end of the regular season, having won twenty out of their thirty games, and trailed Castleford by ten points. But Leeds were masters of saving their best for the Grand Final.

A final game for Leeds, in the championship decider at a sold-out Old Trafford against Castleford of all teams, was a fitting way for Rob and Danny to bow out together. The fact that me, Macy, Maya, his parents and sisters were in the crowd made it even sweeter.

In keeping with the season for Rob, he started on the bench. He was sent on with fifteen minutes to play, the game already won, but I couldn't stop smiling when Rob set up Danny for his second dazzling try, and the fourth for Leeds, as the Rhinos romped to a 24–6 victory.

Danny was the deserved Man of the Match but he insisted that Rob walk up with him to the podium. In an unforgettable moment, their faces lit up with joy, Rob and Danny lifted the Grand Final trophy high in the dark and rainy sky.

I was so happy for Rob, but relieved that his career was finally over.

'I'm a very lucky man to have been involved with a special group of men over seventeen years,' Rob said when he was interviewed on the pitch. 'I've loved every minute of my career. Tonight's a fairy-tale ending for me . . .'

It is often said that a sportsperson dies twice – their first death coming once they can no longer play the game to which they have devoted their life until then. But it was different for Rob. He shared my relief that the struggle to keep proving himself at the age of thirty-five had ended. He looked forward to the rest of his life with us, his family.

Rob still loved rugby; it was all that he really knew in terms of a profession, so it made sense that his transition in retirement would be eased by remaining at Leeds as the Academy head coach. Rob had always enjoyed coaching. Before we were married he had spent three years helping coach some of the junior teams at Ackworth Jaguars, the local club in Pontefract. And when Barrie became the head of youth development at Leeds, after he had retired as a player, he asked Rob to help with some part-time coaching.

This brought some familiar hazards for Barrie because Rob's love of high jinks remained. On one occasion, after Barrie had been tracking the progress of a promising young player for many months, he invited the teenager and his parents to meet him at Headingley. After he collected them from reception, Barrie led the way into his office only to discover that, to his horror, Rob had nipped in a few minutes earlier. Rob had turned around Barrie's laptop so that it faced the door. A new screensaver featured a highly inappropriate image, which Rob had just lifted from the internet. Barrie almost dislocated his shoulder as he dived across the office to slam his laptop shut. It was not the best start to the meeting and Rob felt terrible when the player chose to sign for another club.

Yet, much more than such stunts, Barrie valued Rob's insights and knowledge of the game. When he left the Rhinos and became a pundit at Sky Sports, Barrie often asked to meet for a coffee so that they could discuss the latest tactical intricacies and developments in rugby. Rob would bring his laptop and, as they pored over moves and games, Barrie felt no shame in learning so much from a friend who was ten years younger than him.

He encouraged Rob to eventually seek a full-time coaching career. Barrie later described Rob as 'a wonderful coach who had a great way with the players, especially with the younger ones. He wanted to make sure that the next generation had the best foundation in the game.'

Kevin Sinfield saw the same qualities in Rob and appointed him to his new role. But it's never easy when your whole identity, built for years on your reputation as a player, has to change. It requires a shift in mentality, which came easier to Kev, a more serious man who was used to being in positions of authority as a captain and then as head of rugby at Leeds. Rob found aspects of his coaching job to be stressful. He loved working with young players but some of the more rigorous constraints and administrative responsibilities of the job were harder for him.

I also think Rob was tired and he wanted to spend as much time as he could with us as a family. So he needed to adjust. My belief is that Rob would have done even more outstanding work with the Academy, as he had the right balance of knowledge and empathy, passion and compassion, to have helped hundreds of young players.

In December 2018, Rob and I waited excitedly for the birth of Jackson, our third child and only son. I had gone into labour at thirty-seven weeks with Macy while Maya had arrived a few days past her due date. She'd been born at a midwife-led unit. It was like a home birth in many ways because Rob and I were there with just one midwife who was able to offer gas and air. But there was no other intervention – unless we'd needed assistance with the delivery at the main hospital. All had gone well with Maya and so we planned to follow the same plan with Jackson – the only difference being that our baby boy was seriously late.

I felt great though, and shortly before the big day I was still going to the gym, swimming and even running. But two weeks after my full term the midwife stressed that little Jackson needed a nudge to entice him out into the world.

I went for a sweep – an internal examination where the midwife sweeps a finger around the cervix in an attempt to kick-start labour.

The following night we were in bed and Rob was asleep. I started to feel the familiar twinges but I decided that, rather than waking Rob, I would have a bath. But my relaxing soak did not last long. The contractions began with real intensity. My parents were looking after the girls and so Rob, suddenly wide awake, moved quickly when I said we shouldn't hang around. He rushed me to the midwife unit but I started to really feel I needed to push when we were in the car. I held on but, as we approached the birthing room, I didn't think I was going to make it.

The midwife didn't even have time to take my blood pressure or make any other observations. 'I really need to push,' I gasped.

With her help, and after just three pushes, little Jackson was out.

'It's a boy!' the midwife exclaimed. She then helped Rob cut the cord.

Soon after she had passed our gorgeous boy to me, the midwife said: 'That was so easy. You can come back again.'

Holding Jackson close to me, and resting my back against Rob, I just smiled at her and said, 'No, that's it. We're done now, one hundred per cent.'

I meant it. Our family was complete. Our lives were perfect.

Early the following summer, we had a beautiful routine. In between Rob's coaching and my work as a physio we found just the right balance. Rob was so involved in the lives of the children, and he had such a special relationship with the girls who were by now seven and four, that he often took them to their playgroups while I looked after Jackson.

It gave Rob a real break from his coaching work and, rather than moan about the childcare chores, he loved them.

We were also happy in our house in Pontefract and were caught up with renovations. So we were not even considering moving when, on the way home from work one afternoon, Rob noticed that a house we had previously liked had just come back on the market. It had been built in 2012 and we had wanted to buy it while I was pregnant with Macy. So we were immediately interested when Rob spotted a *For Sale* sign at the bottom of the drive. He called the estate agent and it felt like fate was on our side as the house had only gone on the market that day.

We got the first viewing and were smitten as soon as we walked into the house. We made an offer the next morning – and it was accepted. The sale of our old house also happened quickly and, about four months later, we moved in on a late summer day in September 2019. Rob and I were thrilled, and the girls were jumping around in excitement before they ran through the house and into the big garden outside. Jackson, at only ten months old, slept peacefully while we gazed in wonder at our new home.

Late that night, with boxes still to be unpacked but the kids fast asleep, Rob and I smiled helplessly at each other. We had done it. We had our amazing little family and our dream home.

We had no idea then that, in another three months, Rob would be diagnosed with MND. Our seemingly perfect lives would never be the same again.

8

A Friend Like Kev

Rob was never in denial. He understood the hard truth of his diagnosis; every day he endured the reality that MND had invaded and occupied him. Even while his mind teemed with intelligence and emotion, the disease imprisoned him. It robbed him of speech and movement and left him unable to attend to his basic human needs.

One day, decades before the end of his natural lifespan, it would terminate his life.

Although Rob lived with these facts more graphically than any of us, he really didn't want to talk about them. He preferred to keep smiling because he wanted to find moments of joy in the here and now. He saw no point in moaning or wailing about his fate.

The power of Rob's mentality and positivity came from his years in rugby. Being written off as being too small, too frail, steeled him. Even as a little boy he developed a grit and determination to defy the dismissive predictions and overwhelming odds against him. He learned that, despite the adversity, you could still dream big.

So there was no self-pity in Rob. There were never any

despairing howls of 'Why me?' or 'What have I done to deserve this?' Instead, he still felt grateful for all we had as a family and for each new day he shared with us.

Some days, of course, were really tough. It was always difficult around Christmas or any birthday. Those were the rare times when, quietly, Rob would say to me: 'This might be my last one.'

But he avoided thinking too much about the distressing days that lay ahead. He knew we would gain nothing by worrying about them.

This is not to suggest that Rob refused to think about the future. He sometimes looked ahead but he did so strictly on his terms. As a player he had often used positive visualisation. He imagined breaking a defensive line or haring towards the try line with unstoppable speed. Those euphoric pictures in his head helped him drive through the grind of training. It was as if he was telling himself that all the hard work and constant sacrifice would pay off in the end.

So, trapped in his chair, Rob occasionally allowed his mind to drift away into a dreamy future. He visualised still being with us when Macy and Maya got married. I would push his wheelchair down the aisle, alongside each of the girls, so that he could play a fatherly role on one of the biggest days of their lives. In other imaginary scenarios he saw himself on the touchline, years from now, watching Jackson play rugby as a powerful young man.

I suspect that, deep down, Rob never really believed he would live long enough to see such family milestones. But the hope helped him retain his good cheer, which would be crushed if he focused instead on the grim certainties that were coming.

It was important for me to know Rob's wishes in the dark days ahead. Which medical aids or facilities would he consider using when it became difficult to breathe and swallow? How could we ease his suffering? Where would he want to die? How best might we help him pass away peacefully? What advice would he give me once he was gone, so that I could bring up the children successfully on my own?

It was really difficult, and almost impossible, to have those conversations with Rob.

After the first lockdown in 2020 we had a home visit from Claire Lang, the specialist MND nurse. We had not been able to see any medical professionals in person for months and I was acutely aware of how rapidly Rob's health had deteriorated. His speech was badly slurred and he was unsteady on his feet. He had fallen numerous times and it was becoming harder for him to swallow solid food.

So I asked a serious question in front of Rob. I asked Claire about life expectancy. How much longer did he have left to live?

I can see now that it was poorly worded but I was shocked by Rob's reaction after Claire left. She had avoided giving a specific time frame – but the damage had been done.

Rob was really angry and upset with me. It was a struggle for him to talk but he managed to convey a very clear message. 'Don't ever ask that question again,' Rob said in a ragged voice.

'I promise I won't,' I said, feeling suddenly mortified. 'I'm so sorry, Rob.'

I felt like the worst person in the world and I hated myself for hurting Rob.

He wanted to say more, but it was too difficult to talk. He wanted to tell me how wrong I had been and how I had dashed all the positivity and hope he was trying so hard to preserve.

I, in turn, wanted to explain that I had meant well. It was in my character to be organised and practical but I knew Rob didn't want to hear anything from me right now. He would have walked out of the room if he had been able but, instead, he had to sit silently in his chair, averting his gaze from me. I flitted around in a daze, pretending to tidy up while desperately thinking how I might make Rob feel better. It just made us both feel worse.

I asked Rob if he wanted to watch television and he gave a slight nod. He was still able to turn his head to look at me; but not then. Rob just stared at the flickering screen. He was stewing over my insensitivity and I felt it was best to give him space.

I slipped out into the garden, closing the patio door softly behind me. I walked past the slide, the swing and the trampoline and found a quiet spot near the bottom of the garden. I felt so miserable that I just had to talk to someone. I rang Claire.

I was in floods of tears, and barely responded while Claire tried to calm me. She told me that she understood why I had asked the question and advised me to give Rob time to adjust.

But I knew Rob in a way that she did not. I had seen before how he resisted such conversations and it was plain that he would never talk about these subjects.

I told Claire that I would be all right. I meant it because Rob was too kind to hold it against me for long. He always said we should never go to bed on an argument because Rob was not a man who sulked or held a grudge.

When I went back inside I apologised profusely; Rob softened in front of me. He told me not to worry and he changed the subject to ask when I was picking up the kids. It gave me a chance to natter away about the children and I did my best to keep my tone light and airy.

We never forgot those painful moments but I respected and loved Rob too much to ask that same question in front of him again. Instead, we skirted around the subject, even when we had our annual chat with Dr Lowe, the palliative care consultant from Pinderfields. She would visit us at home so that she could update the hospital's ReSPECT form: Recommended Summary Plan for Emergency Care and Treatment. This little questionnaire was meant to document Rob's wishes.

Some of the questions were very hard to hear. Did he want to be resuscitated, should this be possible, in an end-of-life situation? Would he prefer to die in a hospice or at home?

Dr Lowe and I danced a strange little dance around Rob every year. She appreciated his reluctance to discuss her queries and, as we were dealing with 'respect', we felt compelled to defer to Rob's desire not to engage with the subject. Dr Lowe tried every year but she always withdrew gracefully once Rob made it clear that his views had not changed. He wanted to focus on the best possible life he could have – rather than address ways of dying.

I once asked Dr Lowe if I was being negligent in not pushing

Rob. But she gave me confidence. She was sure that, when the time came, I'd instinctively know what Rob would want.

Rob and I were similar in many ways and very different in others. He had always been happy to settle for an easy life, while I am more highly strung. If something goes wrong, I take it personally; Rob would brush it off as a minor inconvenience.

My desire to have everything mapped out helped whenever I took Rob out of the house. Even a simple visit to the park or an afternoon at the cinema had become a major expedition that required intricate planning. I used to think that it took a lot of organisation to make sure I had everything a toddler needed for a trip. But I had to be much more efficient when getting everything ready for Rob once MND really took hold.

I had to train myself to let certain issues go for Rob's sake. As much as I wanted to have a strategy for every stage of MND, leading to the inevitable end-of-life plan, I let Rob lead the way. We would try to live in the moment. I would face each new problem and rely on my love for Rob to find the right answer.

Dr Jung, the remarkable neurologist leading Rob's care team, was an ally to us both. She told the BBC, in a second documentary, that she and Rob 'have a relationship of trust and mutual respect and lots of laughter in clinic. So it's really lovely, actually, looking after him.'

The documentary cut away to a scene they had filmed when Rob and I visited Dr Jung at Seacroft Hospital. It was a typical interaction between the three of us and began with Dr

Jung turning to Rob to ask: 'So are you using the ventilator overnight?'

As it was easier for Rob, I answered with a smile: 'Intermittently. I don't think he particularly likes having it on so we tend to do it sort of one night on, one night off.'

Rob then responded. 'It gets uncomfortable for my big nose,' he said, using his voice app to reply.

Dr Jung laughed. 'Did it get broken many times?'

'No, I think it's on his grandad's side,' I said. 'Is it the Bateman nose? I think so.'

Dr Jung asked another important question. 'How's the eating and drinking?'

We waited for Rob's reply: 'I'm never full.'

'I can't fill him at the minute,' I admitted, 'despite the puddings and custard.'

Dr Jung spoke gently to Rob: 'I know in the past you've said no to assisted nutrition discussions?'

'No, don't waste your time,' Rob answered, with the robotic sound of his voice missing the wry humour in his reply.

Dr Jung laughed. 'These responses get better and better every time.'

'I was waiting for that one,' I said.

'Right, let's have a look at you,' Dr Jung said to Rob. 'I'm just going to get my little tendon hammer.'

In a more personal observation, Dr Jung told the film-makers that 'motor neurone disease is an extremely cruel condition'.

She was then filmed testing Rob in a visual examination. 'One finger,' she said, holding it in the air. 'Keep your head steady, follow this with your eyes. Don't move your head . . . don't move your head. Look up. And down here.'

Dr Jung chided him playfully. 'No, you're moving your head, Rob.'

I agreed: 'He's cheating.'

Rob was always too smart for us. In one of our earliest meetings Dr Jung had also tried to persuade him that he needed to confront the uncomfortable realities that would be so problematic in the future. She appealed to the sportsman in Rob. Surely he had planned for future matches as a rugby player?

Rob gave her a knowing smile. 'Well,' he said, 'I always planned for the next game. I didn't plan for six games ahead.'

We laughed helplessly then, Dr Jung and I, knowing we had been outflanked by my canny husband.

Rob's deterioration was marked in every aspect of his life. In 2020 it became increasingly hard for him to lift his leg because his muscles had weakened, and so I began to help him climb the stairs to bed every night. That soon led to me picking him up from behind so that I could carry him upstairs. It was difficult and worrying because I didn't want the two of us to fall backwards and end up in a broken heap at the bottom of the stairs.

He used a Zimmer frame downstairs, which did not dignify a former professional sportsman in his late thirties. It resembled a little trolley, which he could use as a seat when he became tired. But we couldn't use that for long as it soon reached a point where Rob's balance was so bad that he would just fall down.

In 2023 we made the decision to move Rob permanently downstairs. A specialist profiling bed had been loaned to us as it would be much more comfortable for Rob. I still slept upstairs, which felt very lonely, but I knew Rob's nights would be more peaceful without me coming in and out, switching on the lights or turning over in bed.

Rob never told me how this enforced separation made him feel at night. He rarely got upset and did not often share his true feelings. He always just said, 'I'm OK.' But I suspect that he, too, found it painful that we would never sleep in the same bed together again.

There are so many ways to show love and care. Rob and I found new ways to deepen our relationship, even if so much was underpinned by the most basic human needs to sleep, eat, drink and go to the toilet. Once Rob could no longer feed himself we had to change the kind of food he ate. He became increasingly reliant on soft food and we needed to be flexible just as Rob was becoming more rigid in both his movement and thinking.

Rob only wanted me or his mum to feed him and, as the months passed, we learned that his jaws could clamp shut on a metal spoon. He would bite down so hard, without meaning to do so, and he once lost a crown. We had to switch to wooden and plastic spoons.

My biggest concern was trying to make sure that I could get enough food, and nutrients, into Rob's system. Weight loss was a constant worry.

His swallowing became so compromised that he could no

179

longer even drink from a straw, which had been his chosen way for nearly a year. We resorted to sealed cups, which resembled baby beakers. If I was in the kitchen, the kids would often call me when Rob needed to be moved or taken to the toilet. But if he was thirsty they could just tilt the cup and gently pour the drink into his mouth.

There were regular toilet issues because the painkillers and his inability to move meant he often became constipated and needed laxatives. We also sometimes had the opposite problem with incontinence and so I became quite used to enemas as well. People might think this would be hard. But how can it be when you are looking after someone you love with all your heart? It also helped that my medical background meant there was no squeamishness on my part.

Rob was great. He was a proud man, and I know it hurt him that he had to rely on me to such an extent, but I also loved the fact that he was not embarrassed or ashamed of our normal bodily functions. Rob, after all, was the kind of character who would walk around the Rhinos dressing room completely naked while singing a Michael Jackson song or telling a joke. I remember that, years ago, a Sky television crew had been allowed into the changing room. They had to cut away quickly when a naked man was caught on camera. It had to be Rob.

He was not shy when he had to be showered – although he again insisted that he would only be cleaned by either me or his mum. At least he agreed that Irene could be helped by our brother-in-law, Mike, as it was not easy for his mum to support

Rob on her own. So, for the most part, we coped well in the bathroom. There were just a few occasions when I'd put him on the toilet and turn away for twenty seconds. Next thing there would be an almighty thud as Rob toppled straight off the toilet.

It was hard to pick Rob up from the floor and I would ask the girls for help if they were at home: 'Can you pull Daddy's trousers up for me, Macy?' or 'Can you straighten Daddy's knees for me, Maya?'

We learn from our mistakes and I soon made sure never to turn away from Rob in the loo.

During our early years with MND we managed to go away on a few holidays. After the first Covid lockdown, we went on a staycation Disney cruise. The five of us drove with my parents, my brother and his family and my aunt and uncle to Liverpool, where we took a Disney theme-boat that sailed around the Irish Sea. We dressed in Disney costumes and the kids all had Disney suitcases. I wore giant Minny Mouse ears. Rob, being such a Disney fanatic, loved it.

We had a few more weekend breaks around the UK – going to Alton Towers, Center Parcs and Aysgarth in the Yorkshire Dales – and in August 2022 we braved a trip to Gran Canaria with my parents. But Rob found the plane journey and all the travel hard to bear. He was exhausted by the time we got home. We knew then he would never be able to leave the country again.

His world had shrunk even more, but Rob kept smiling and finding joy close to home.

*

Kevin Sinfield contributed to that joy in extraordinary ways. Every year he pushed his body to brutal extremes to support Rob, highlight the plight of thousands of MND patients and to raise millions of pounds in our ongoing battle against the disease.

It was only meant to be one challenge, to help Rob and our family, in December 2020. After a grim and surreal year, in which our lives had been turned inside out while the pandemic had decimated the world, Kev was worried about meeting a figure that he and Rob thought we needed to offset any lost income from coaching.

So Kev set himself an incredible challenge. He decided to run seven marathons in seven days with the aim of raising £77,777 for Rob. The heavy emphasis on all those sevens was a tribute to the shirt number that Rob had worn throughout his seventeen-year-long career.

Once Kev sets his mind on a task there is no stopping him. He went through hell for Rob. It was often bitingly cold and rainy, and it even snowed on the third morning. By the time he crossed the finish line after his seventh marathon he had already raised £1.2 million. The figure did not stop there either and by then Rob and I had decided that we would share the money with the MND Association and other charities. An astonishing total of £2.7 million was donated.

Of all the challenges that Kev has gone on to complete, I think that the first one was the hardest emotionally. In subsequent years, Kev has been accompanied by an army of supporters and the roads have been thronged with people cheering him on. But most of his marathon-running in 2020 was very lonely.

When Kev began his first run on Tuesday 1 December we were still in the second lockdown. It had begun on 31 October when Boris Johnson said we needed to return to isolation to prevent a 'medical and moral disaster for the NHS'.

Kev simply ran on and on, up and down the empty roads, as his suffering intensified with each new marathon. He couldn't sleep much at night, as his body ached and his mind raced. There were days where he was either shivering helplessly or in serious danger of overheating.

'Throughout all the runs, at different stages, I'd be welling up and choking up,' Kev said later. 'It was so emotional because it's really difficult to see Rob now, compared to where we were twelve months ago. Rob's thirty-eight, he's got three young kids and nobody deserves it because this is the cruellest disease. I know there're some horrific diseases out there but to see what MND does to families, to see the strain it puts on them, is so difficult. It's a horrible, horrible disease.

'Rob's kids are great. They've got big smiles on their faces. Lindsey is always smiling, she's been so strong. And every time I see Rob, he's got a big smile on his face and that twinkle in his eye so you absolutely know what he's thinking. We still laugh at the stupidest jokes and we're constantly reminding each other of things on text or when I see him.'

The lockdown eased and the most draconian restrictions had been lifted by day five of Kev's challenge. People were able to turn out in Leeds as Kev approached Headingley. We were waiting for him. I held Jackson while Macy and Maya danced in excitement around me. Next to us,

Rob grinned in his wheelchair, which was held by Geoff and Irene.

We watched Kev turn the corner and run past the new mural of Rob near the stadium. Kev veered across the road so that he could bump fists with Rob, whose face, looking up at his friend, was a picture of rapture.

'I had to carry on running then,' Kev said later. 'I wasn't letting you see me cry again.'

Kev looked back. As he ran, he raised his right hand and waved to Rob.

There was no chance of Kev containing his tears when, after finishing that marathon, he embraced a beaming Rob.

Kev said that the next day, and the sixth marathon, 'was the toughest by a mile. Some of it was because of the cumulative fatigue, and not sleeping, while parts of my body were in pain. But you could feel the emotion it took out of us after marathon five, to see him and then to have a cuddle with Rob. There was never a moment where I forgot why we were doing it – but to actually see Rob at the end of day five absolutely hammered it home.'

Maya kept us laughing as she told Kev: 'You're nearly as fast as my dad, but not quite . . .'

We were overwhelmed by all that Kev had done for us but gratified, too, that he widened the focus to include all families affected by the disease. Each afternoon, following the completion of another marathon, Kev would talk on Zoom to people with MND. It deepened his understanding of the condition and, more importantly, gave emotional sustenance to the men and women dealing with the catastrophe of MND every day of their lives.

For too long, they had been ignored or forgotten. Kev made sure that they were finally noticed as his marathon exploits lit up the news channels and social media.

'I'm busted and broken now, but it's what mates do,' Kev said. 'They look after each other.'

Rob responded, through his voice app, by saying to Kev: 'You continue to inspire and make me never want to give in. Like you I will take one step at a time. Maybe there isn't a finish line for me but I'll keep on going.'

He paused and then added a simple truth: 'Everyone needs a friend like Kev.'

Kev's next two challenges were even more gruelling. In November 2021, while raising more than a million pounds for MND charities, he ran 104 miles in twenty-four hours. His long and arduous journey took him from Leicester to Headingley. The most moving moments came at the very end when Macy ran the last mile with Kev – who looked drunk with fatigue. He was in a very dark place as sleep deprivation and a lack of proper training had almost unravelled him.

The timing of the run had been all wrong. Kev had started a new job as a rugby union coach with the Leicester Tigers three and a half months earlier. He left home at 4am most mornings, to get to training in Leicester, and he was juggling the demands of work with all he was trying to do for people with MND. His training routine was much more haphazard than a year earlier and so he was in trouble during that twenty-four-hour slog.

But Kev said Macy helped him. She could tell that he was struggling and so before she joined him she paused and then gave him an encouraging smile, which said so much. Together, they completed the last mile. Kev was blown away by her emotional intelligence at such a young age.

'I don't know when I'll be able to run again,' Kev told the BBC soon after the finish. 'Rob knows how much we love and care about him. For those really dark moments, you have to think about Rob. We wanted a battle, and we got one.'

Rob's dad, Geoff, said: 'While we all knew he would do it, the main thing is that Kevin takes care of himself. The money is great but nowhere as important as Kevin's health.'

A year later, Kev was back with his latest challenge. In November 2022 he raised the stakes again by running seven ultra-marathons in seven days. This meant he ran twenty-seven miles, or forty-three kilometres, a day. Kev started his challenge at Scotland's Murrayfield ground in Edinburgh on a Sunday morning and finished it the following Saturday afternoon at Old Trafford. He smashed his target of £777,777 and the money raised sailed past £1 million again.

'Our country cares,' an exhausted Kev said on the Old Trafford pitch during the half-time break at the men's Rugby League World Cup final. 'It cares about people who need help. And the MND community need us. They need support, they need love and we've got to find a cure.'

*

We were amazed yet again when we learned that the inaugural Rob Burrow Leeds Marathon would be held in May 2023 and all the proceeds were to be donated to charities, including the MND Association. Rob and I decided that we would both attempt our first marathon. I'd run it alongside my brother, Mark, and our friend Josh Taylor, while Rob would be pushed around the course in his wheelchair by Kev.

It felt very serious when the organisers, Run For All, told us our race numbers. More than 12,000 runners had entered and I would set off in a bib marked with the number 1. 'No pressure then,' I joked to Rob who had been given his favourite number 7.

I had run for years and had always loved it. So I trained as much as I could, in between looking after Rob, and one Sunday in January I went for a twenty-mile run. I was delighted with my time of three hours and seven minutes. It meant that, if I matched that pace in the actual marathon, I would have another hour and fifty-three minutes to complete the last six miles. Even if I had to walk it, I would finish in under five hours – which was my humble target.

I felt really good and, the following Tuesday, I went swimming and then did an eight-mile run. As I neared the end, cruising down our road and just a few minutes from home, I felt pain in my knee. It was a little concerning but I thought it was just a niggle that needed a few days of rest. But time was ticking and so I went out the following week for a long run. I thought I would ease myself back in and run for sixteen, rather than twenty, miles. My knee hurt most of the way and, by the thirteen-mile mark, I'd been reduced to a hobble. I had to stop and limp slowly home.

An elderly gent even came up and asked if I needed any help. I reassured him that I just had a sore knee. But an MRI scan eventually showed damage to the cartilage at the back of the patella, which is known as the chondromalacia patella. It was my body's way of telling me that I'd overtrained. There were nine weeks left to the marathon and the knee had to be rested for a minimum of five weeks.

I lost a lot of fitness and both Rob and I felt a little uncertain as to what lay in store for us when we turned up on the start line on Sunday 14 May 2023. I felt horribly unprepared for my run. But I thought I had prepped Rob well for his race and had chosen his outfit carefully. As he was so thin and frail, he felt the cold deep down in his bones. So I put him in a thermal vest and covered it with a big fleece. His running vest went on top of the fleece and I told Rob he would be nice and snug in the open air. I had no apprehension about Rob because he would be looked after by Superman, or Kev as we still called him.

The day turned out to be a scorcher – really hot and sunny. When we made the halfway point of a very hilly course, Mark asked me if I had remembered to pack some sunscreen for Rob. I hadn't and I felt terrible. I had no way of finding Rob and Kev as we had been separated hours earlier.

At that stage I was also struggling with my knee, a few blisters and the long, unforgiving hills. But the atmosphere was amazing and that kept me going. People were giving me high fives and shouting out my name in encouragement. It was lovely but also really hard as I was not in great shape. I bit down on the pain and thought that, if Rob could put up with discomfort every hour of every day, I could withstand a sore knee and a few blisters.

I also knew that once I finished I would have raised £110,000 for the Leeds Hospital charity fund – flying past my initial target of £7,777. So nothing was going to stop me crossing the line. I made it to the end and, even though I was disappointed with my time of five hours and three minutes, I was happy to see the family.

Maya soon had me laughing through my sweaty heavy breathing. 'Mum,' she asked seriously, 'why did so many really old people run past you?'

My laughter faded as soon as I saw poor Rob. He looked terrible after an excruciating ordeal. He and Kev had finished more than half an hour ahead of me and, just before the end, they had shared an almost unbearably poignant moment. Kev had stopped the wheelchair. He'd bent down to unbuckle Rob and then, with great tenderness, he had lifted his friend out of the chair. Kev then carried Rob over the finishing line.

A photograph of that moment would circulate on social media and eventually make headlines. It was an image so inspiring that it came to symbolise Rob and Kev's friendship and their fundraising efforts for MND.

But we had totally underestimated the demands of the marathon on Rob's body. Every bump in the road shuddered through him and the wheelchair had felt like a suntrap. He was boiling in all the layers I had chosen for him and his face looked hot and flushed.

Most of all he was exhausted. He wanted to be put to bed as soon as we got home. It would take him another two days to recover and I could see how much he had suffered while the marathon in his name raised just over £1,770,000. At least the presence of a couple of lucky 7s, in yet another staggering haul for MND, made Rob smile.

Six weeks later Rob picked up a cold, which he couldn't shake. There were also complications because even the simple feat of coughing was beyond him. For a healthy person, a cough can loosen and clear the chest of phlegm and all the associated gunk that comes with the common cold. Rob did not have that luxury. His chest and lungs were clogged, so when we called the doctor out, he was immediately prescribed some antibiotics.

I blame myself now because Rob hadn't been eating much for a couple of days and he looked malnourished. In hindsight it seems obvious that I should have called the doctor much earlier.

Rob insisted that he was well enough to do a Zoom meeting with Kev, as they were working on a children's book, but he agreed that he should rest in bed before they began. He got through the meeting but immediately asked to be put back to bed. It was so unlike Rob.

I left him to sleep and, feeling worried, picked up the children from school.

In the early evening he seemed a little better and I lifted him up from the bed and settled him in his chair to watch some television. He didn't want to eat anything but I fed the kids and, after the usual rushing around, got them down to bed.

Rob looked far worse when I came downstairs. My concern turned to trepidation – especially when I asked if he wanted me to call the NHS helpline 111. Rob said 'yes', an answer he usually resisted.

The woman on 111 listened carefully as I explained Rob's symptoms and mentioned his laboured breathing. She said that a doctor would call me as soon as possible.

During that video call I noticed the alarm on the doctor's face when she looked at Rob. She said that she had concerns about his breathing because his respiratory rate seemed quite high. A chill cut through me when she said: 'I think we should send an ambulance to get Rob to hospital.'

She was obviously right but that certainty made me feel very frightened for the first time in the long three and a half years of caring for Rob. A terrifying thought made the breath catch at the back of my throat. I couldn't say the words out loud but they reverberated in my head: *What if Rob goes into hospital and never comes out?*

I kissed Rob on his damp and fevered brow and then phoned his mum. I packed a small bag for Rob and prepared him for our departure, still wondering if it would be permanent for him.

My heart was racing. Everything moved so quickly.

Irene arrived, followed soon after by the ambulance. I rushed out to speak to the paramedics. I needed to make sure they did not turn on their blue lights and wake the kids. The thought of them also being frightened so late at night was almost too much too bear.

The paramedics came in quietly and quickly. After examining

Rob they said we needed to get him comfortable in hospital. There was such kindness in them too because, when they heard that I would follow in the van that we used to transport Rob and his wheelchair, one of the paramedics made a lovely suggestion. He said that he and Rob would travel with me. I could drive while he looked after Rob. That little gesture calmed me and made me feel a little less alone.

The wonderful Irene would look after Macy, Maya and Jackson if they woke in the night.

'I'll be back to take them to school in the morning,' I promised.

'Don't worry about that now, love,' Irene said soothingly.

But I did. It was Macy's transition day and I knew how important it was that I drove her to the senior school where she would be starting Year 7 a few months from then.

Rob needed me, though, and I was so relieved that there were no blue lights to cast disturbing shadows across the kids' bedroom windows. I drew in a couple of deep breaths to steady myself. I just needed to drive safely to Pinderfields in Wakefield so that Rob could be saved.

A little convoy, with the yellow ambulance leading our black van, drove quietly away from our slumbering house. We moved into the dark night and towards an unknown fate.

Seven hours later, just after 6am, I gently opened the front door. Irene was waiting for me as she had not slept much either. I had been up all night but at least I could tell her that Rob was stable and asleep at Pinderfields.

They had taken him to the respiratory high-dependency unit and, after an examination, the hospital had given him a chest X-ray and a series of blood tests. Medication had followed and, at around three in the morning, an exhausted Rob had finally drifted off. I sat at his bedside, watching his emaciated chest rise and fall. I then looked with overwhelming love at his grey and sunken face covered in an oxygen mask.

Rob had pneumonia. It's a serious condition for anyone but, in the case of a patient with MND, it can be terminal.

Irene shared my deep concern but I reassured her. The doctors were positive. They believed that the right antibiotics would fight the pneumonia that left Rob looking more depleted than I had ever seen him. The oxygen and round-the-clock medical care would also help.

We agreed that Irene should slip home before the kids woke to avoid our having to answer any questions about their dad. Rob's door was closed and he usually slept until an hour or so after I returned from the morning school run.

I had just enough time to shower and change before it was time to get the children up. Maya and Jackson were very sleepy but Macy had been awake for a while. She looked pale with nerves.

Transition day is a big deal for any boy or girl because it is a first little taste of senior school which, when you are only ten or eleven, belongs to the big bad world outside. It was harder for Macy too because she was not going to the same new school as any of her friends; all her pals from primary school had chosen to go elsewhere. But Macy had set her heart on the school we would be driving to in the next hour. She felt it would be the best school for her and Rob and I were so proud of her for making such a mature decision. It would have been very easy to have stuck with the pack but Macy is as brave as she is intelligent.

Her courage, however, briefly dipped. I hugged her tight and promised her that it would all work out.

As I felt her arms wrap around me, I knew that I had done the right thing in being with her that morning. But I had also felt desolate and guilty leaving the hospital. How could I walk away from Rob when he was so ill?

I felt torn inside.

There was no time left for conflicted feelings. My parents arrived to pick up Jackson and Maya to take them to their nursery and Year 2 class. We were out the door in a rush as Maya turned around to shout: 'Bye, Daddy!'

Macy's face broke into her first smile of the day. 'Bye, Dad,' she called out.

And then, in a heart-rending chorus, the girls looked at Rob's closed door and shouted together: 'Love you!'

A fresh wave of guilt washed over me. It felt as if I was lying to them. I almost wanted to stop and explain the truth. But how could Macy face her transition day if she knew that her dad was seriously ill in hospital?

I kissed Maya and Jackson goodbye and told Mum and Dad that I would be in touch later. They knew that I would be calling from Pinderfields and so, with sombre smiles full of love, they nodded before brightening so that they could wish Macy good luck.

Macy was quiet in the car but I spoke positively about how certain we were that she was making the right decision. I had no doubt that she would love the school and make new friends.

She nodded and looked ahead. I kept talking and turned on the radio to keep the mood nice and normal as if it were just an ordinary school morning. Macy still looked nervous as we parked near the school. 'It's going to be great,' I said. 'I promise. C'mon, I'll walk you in . . .'

I knew I couldn't reach out to hold her hand, as we were on our way to 'big school', but I walked close to Macy and smiled at everyone we passed.

'Thanks, Mum,' she said softly as she lifted her head and we walked through the school gates.

Macy was beaming when I picked her up that afternoon. Words tumbled happily from her as she told me all about her day, from the teachers to the girls she had met. Everything had gone well and she could hardly stop smiling.

We had been talking for almost ten minutes when, on our way to pick up Maya and Jackson from my parents, Macy looked across at me.

'Mum,' she said searchingly, 'are you okay? Has something happened?'

It was typical of Macy, who has such empathy and insight, to pick up on my mood. I had hidden it that morning but, knowing that she had done so well with her transition day, my facade had cracked.

I could have broken down but I knew how important it was that I stayed strong for Macy, Maya and Jackson.

The girls looked worried, and Jackson was confused, when I explained that their dad was in hospital. It felt important to be truthful while reassuring them that their dad was getting special care. The doctors had also told me that they thought he could come home in five days.

The kids wanted to see Rob and we spent that late afternoon at Pinderfields. He smiled so happily when he saw them burst into the room and they chattered away cheerfully to him.

But it was also a shock. The girls, in particular, were upset when we left. They had never seen their dad looking so fragile and weak.

'Is Daddy going to die?' Maya asked in the car.

Macy turned to look closely at me. 'Is he, Mum?'

It was so hard hearing my children ask such questions. I spoke as honestly as I could. I told them that I really believed their dad would come home. They weren't to worry because I was going to look after him better than ever.

'We all will,' Maya exclaimed.

Her big sister, having come through a testing day, nodded intently. 'We'll help you, Mum,' Macy said. 'We really will.'

A few days after Rob came home, and while he was sleeping peacefully, I had a follow-up telephone consultation with Dr Lowe, the palliative care consultant at Pinderfields. In the course of that conversation I asked her the question that I could not say in front of Rob. How long did he have left to live?

Dr Lowe reminded me gently that Rob had been very poorly in hospital. She said it might be a matter of weeks or, knowing Rob, he could still be with us months from now. He was such a fighter that perhaps he could make it to Christmas. But the end was closing in on us.

I was bereft, but unsurprised. When Rob was still at Pinderfields I had met with Dr Lowe and the respiratory care consultant. We discussed the painful subject of whether Rob would ever allow the implantation of a PEG (percutaneous endoscopic gastrostomy) which, through surgery, allows a feeding tube to give the body the nutrients and sustenance it needs to survive. Rob was struggling to eat and had to rely on soups and other liquid-based foods. He desperately needed a PEG.

But there were complications. Was Rob strong enough to withstand surgery? If we couldn't feed him properly, would he ever be ready for the operation?

It was inevitable that Rob would eventually lose the capacity to swallow. He would then be reduced to a husk in his chair. The idea that Rob would effectively starve to death terrified me.

I had read about political prisoners who went on hunger strike and refused all food and water. They were healthy when their strike began and some of them could survive for sixty or seventy days before death finally came. But, until that merciful release, their suffering was excruciating.

I was not sure I could survive seeing Rob endure such

trauma – even if his already skeletal frame meant that his agony would be shorter.

I told Dr Lowe and her colleague that, personally, I had wanted Rob to have the PEG fitted months before. But he'd made it clear, as he had always done, that he would not consider it. Accepting a feeding tube would be proof that he had finally surrendered to MND.

Rob, even now, was not willing to give up. He would keep fighting until the very end.

I had always respected Rob's wishes, and I always will. MND had stripped him of so much. I was not willing to take away his freedom to choose how he would live and die.

I was ready to fight on with Rob, for as many days, weeks and months that we had left.

9

The Password Is Hero

The long winter dragged on, but Rob and I were still full of warmth and light. Monday 26 February 2024 was the start of another week: the kids were at school and I'd be back working at the hospital in Leeds early the following morning. Rob had slept late, until around ten as usual. I'd then taken him to the toilet, given him a wash and a very small breakfast – he just wanted one of his nutritional shakes – but he seemed cheerful and comfortable as I settled him in his chair so that he could watch another episode of his latest series on Netflix.

'Are you okay if I nip out and have thirty minutes at the gym, Rob?' I asked.

He gave me a big grin. It had become too exhausting to use his Eyegaze machine for ordinary conversation because it was a piece of technology that required him to use his eyes to identify individual letters on the screen and then, slowly, build words to formulate an answer. So Rob saved it for when he wanted to ask me to do something. Instead we had come up with a really basic method of communication. When I asked Rob a question all he needed to do was to move his eyes to the left to say 'yes' or shift them to the right for 'no'.

I watched his eyes move to the left. As always, I double-checked. 'I'll be back in less than an hour, but are you sure?'

Rob was always so patient with me and, once more, he looked to the left to say yes.

I kissed him and made sure that his show started at the right episode. I ran around, picking up my gym gear, bag and car keys, conscious again of how easily I flitted around the house while Rob remained locked inside his motionless body.

'Is there anything else you need, darling?' I asked, knowing it might be something as simple as me scratching his itchy nose or making him more comfortable in his chair. He smiled again, moving his gaze to the right.

I leant down and stole another kiss. 'I love you,' I said.

Of course Rob remained silent but I felt his love for me all over again. 'I won't be long,' I promised. 'Back soon and text me anytime.'

It was time to get going: any free slots away from the house and caring for Rob were so fleeting and so rare.

I left at 11.35, made it to the gym, worked out for half an hour, and was just walking back to the car when my phone pinged at 12.25. I read the message from Rob: *Could I please have a coffee from McDonald's, darling?*

I kept walking while smiling and texting: *Go on, seeing as it's you,* I replied.

I added a little winking emoji and our favourite three words: *I love you.*

Rob sent a thumbs-up before, a minute later, another message came from him: *I've just bit my lip.*

Sometimes, after Rob yawned, his teeth clamped down on his lip as his mouth closed. He couldn't always control the muscles in his face and so, when this happened, he needed me or one of the girls to gently prise open his mouth to free his lip. The consultant had offered him Botox injections but Rob made a joke about not being a Hollywood star and so he was prescribed Baclofen, a skeletal muscle relaxant used by people with multiple sclerosis or spinal problems. It alleviates muscle spasms, but Rob's problem was different and Baclofen didn't help him much.

There were so many little struggles for Rob. He wore a collar to support his neck but we could never quite find the right one for him. He didn't like the hard collars because they tilted his head back. While they offered more head control they were so rigid that they made him feel as if he was suffocating when dribbling from his mouth. The smaller, softer collars were more forgiving, but they gave only minimal head control.

The chair was also difficult. While the one we'd chosen was more comfortable for him to sit on than other models, it rubbed against his ears and left little weeping sores. We were always fighting against something. He could use a machine that helped his breathing by removing the carbon dioxide but Rob didn't like it because, again, he felt as if he was suffocating.

There is never an ideal scenario for an MND patient. It's a constant trade-off where one form of relief provides another dash of discomfort.

As I raced home to free Rob's lip, I felt the consuming agony of his situation all over again. The paralysis tested his spirit every hour of every day and yet, somehow, Rob remained positive despite his overwhelming helplessness. How could I be depressed or self-pitying when I saw Rob's refusal to give in to the frozen ruin of his body?

My biggest daily concern for Rob was that we were not managing to give him enough nutrition. He was painfully thin and frail, and it was a constant battle to feed him. Rob had little appetite as it was too difficult for him to swallow even mashed-up food. Where once he would have relished eating puréed cottage pie followed by sponge pudding and custard turned to mush in the blender, it had become easier for Rob to just rely on his shakes. He had an app that recorded his daily calorie count but I worried more and more that the shakes couldn't give him the full nourishment he needed.

Of course Rob just smiled when, having flown through the front door, I liberated his lip from the grip of his teeth. His eyes moved left when I asked him if he was okay and I was relieved to see him enjoying his coffee. I chattered away about my session at the gym, the horrible weather outside and our plans for the weekend with the kids.

Rob couldn't answer, but that's why his texts meant so much to me. I still got a little thrill when he called me 'darling' or told me he loved me. It was typical of Rob to wake up long after I was home from taking the kids to school and, using his eyes, text me to say: *Good morning, darling. You have a good night's sleep? If you could please proceed with the shower to 12:30?*

By 2024, the messages didn't always make complete sense – but I would pop my head round the corner, say a cheery hello, give him a hug and a kiss and soon work out what he meant about the shower.

He could also be totally coherent in his texts and say: 'Hope you're having an excellent day and thanks again for your help. I love you' or 'You have a good day, darling, we love you so much.'

But as winter turned to a sodden spring his messages became muddled. 'Sorry, I have to come home tonight, I'll be absolutely' one text in April 2024 said before it ran out of steam. Another suggested, without any accompanying context, 'We have to be careful about the car. The garage, we absolutely don't want to be driving this.'

On other occasions he was less confused but I could still tell he was struggling to text: 'I'm hoping that you are able for you having a lovely day and we love you so much.'

His messages meant the world to me, and I will always keep them, but from May 2024 Rob could no longer text me. We had taken him to have his eyes tested but I knew that it was just too much for him to message me.

It made me feel how deeply I missed the conversations that had filled our house four and a half years before. I missed hearing Rob ask if he could do anything to help or telling me I looked beautiful in a new dress. I missed hearing him steady me when I was worried about one of the kids or feeling tired after a long day of difficult consultations at work. I missed hearing him kidding around with the girls or speaking softly to Jackson. I missed hearing him laugh.

I felt lonely – but it was nothing compared to Rob's isolation in a prison of his own silence and stillness.

He was locked into MND's cell of solitary confinement. Rob might have been able to see us and hear us but his inability to move, to talk and eventually even to eat sealed his seclusion. He had been given a life sentence, but it was a death sentence too.

But Rob showed me how to live. He found pleasure and hope in small moments. When the kids came home and told him excitedly about their day at school, or how they had done at drama or gymnastics or football, Rob was captivated. He went to every activity of theirs that he could and pride and happiness poured out of him when watching them.

Instead of being bitter and resentful about the cruel way his life had come to a halt, Rob thought how lucky he was to have me, the kids, his parents and sisters, my family and all his friends. He was thankful for all that remained. And so he made me appreciate all I had. I still had Rob and I was just as grateful for the miracle of our three happy children.

He made me think of others who were so much less fortunate than us – and far less well known than Rob. I had met full-time carers who had neither the money nor family support to boost them when times became hard. They were almost as trapped and isolated as their loved ones, who could no longer carry out even the most basic human tasks for themselves.

It was much easier for me, in comparison, as I had my parents and Rob's family to help. Our place in the public eye also meant that people went out of their way to show support to us. And no other MND patient had quite the same public outpouring of love, which bolstered Rob.

He made me feel lucky to have loved him for twenty-six years and to be in a position where I could care for him. I also valued the happy and fun times we had shared since we were just kids of fifteen. Obviously, I wished we could have looked forward to another twenty-six years, and more, together. But the tender life lessons Rob gave to me meant that I, following his lead, came to appreciate all that we had once had – however much time we had left – and to live in the moment. I still laughed and smiled with Rob when we watched the kids thriving. I still felt utterly alive as I tried to do the very best for them and for Rob.

But MND is brutal. It ravages its victims physically, mentally and emotionally. Even Rob, with his mighty heroism, finally began to buckle. In mid-April 2024 he found the resolve to type me a message. It came out of the blue and my heart cracked a little as I read the seven words Rob had texted:

I'm finding it hard to fight MND.

I walked across to Rob, feeling the magnitude of the moment when I saw he had become tearful. It was the first time he had cried in years.

Bending down, I held him close, kissed him and told him that I understood. But I knew that he didn't want me to pity him so I tried to lift his spirits. 'I know things are getting harder for you, Rob,' I said. 'But you've done so well. Keep fighting, darling, keep going. You've always been so positive for us, so I want to be positive for you.'

Rob's eyes swam with desperate tears. 'Hold on, darling,' I urged, knowing how futile my words sounded in the surrounding silence.

We were alone in the house, with the kids at school, and I was shaken. Apart from the first twenty-four hours following his diagnosis back in December 2019, it was the only time Rob had actually admitted he was struggling. His determination and strength floored me every day but, suddenly, I was worried. I could see how worn out he looked.

'We'll keep going, Rob, okay?' I said, my voice thick with emotion.

I took a step back to look at him properly. My hands rested lightly on his emaciated shoulders. 'Okay, darling?' I asked, seeking to reassure us both.

Rob's pale blue eyes brimmed with anguish. But he knew I needed an answer and, after a long pause, he turned his gaze to the left. And then I felt my breaking heart soar when he smiled.

The signs of deterioration increased with each passing day in May. I had arranged for my mum and dad to have the kids stay over so that Rob and I could visit Ed Slater, the former rugby union player, who had been diagnosed with MND in July 2022. But Rob was too ill to travel. We had to send our apologies to Ed so that Rob could rest.

On Sunday 12 May, at the Rob Burrow Leeds Marathon, the plan had been that Kev Sinfield would run almost the entire 26.2 miles before he scooped up Rob in his arms. They would then finish the last 10 metres together as Kev carried Rob. But a few days before the marathon Rob told me that he didn't feel well enough for that ordeal as his fragile body would jar with every step Kev ran.

Rob still attended the race and he smiled at the end when Kev crossed the line and came straight over to us. Maya and Macy stood proudly behind their dad's wheelchair while I knelt down and Kev crouched to be eye-level with Rob. I had run the half-marathon, with little training, but I was proud of Rob rather than myself.

Fourteen thousand people had turned out to run and raise money for MND and other charities. But I also knew how hard the day was for Rob and he was shattered when we got home.

I asked him if he wanted to go to bed. His glassy eyes looked to the left. There was no need to double-check his answer and Rob was soon in bed, looking ghostly and depleted.

Over the next two weeks he spent large chunks of each day dozing in his chair. My parents had noticed his deterioration and, where once Rob had been so engaged and did his best to answer their questions with his eyes, he now often stared into space without showing any sign that he had heard them.

I began to prepare myself for the end. But I had no idea how many weeks, or months, we had left. A weight of sadness pressed down on me, especially when I was alone, but I tried hard to fight it. It was important for me to keep going, to try to look sunny and cheerful for Rob and the kids. I wanted Macy, Maya and Jackson to feel as normal as possible, for as long as possible. The terrible abnormality of losing their dad was coming.

Angela Elsworth, my lovely friend, texted me on Wednesday 22 May. Her surprise message lifted me. She and her friends were going to see Take That on Friday night in Middlesbrough. Angela had a spare ticket and asked if I would like to join them. She knew how much I'd loved Take That as a girl – Mark Owen was my favourite member of the group. Rob was always amused at how I had been quietly smitten during that early teenage crush.

Reminiscing about those days of carefree innocence felt like a break from real life and the idea of going to the gig with Angela was very appealing. Middlesbrough was just over an hour away and so I could still pick up the kids from school, give them their tea, drop them off at my mum's and be back from the gig soon after midnight. But I didn't want to leave Rob unless he was happy to spend the night at his parents' house. So, barefoot (as I always was in the house), I padded from the kitchen to the front room where Rob looked drowsy in his chair. I checked whether he needed a drink and if he was comfortable and then asked if it would be okay to go to the gig.

Rob looked to the left. I couldn't help but ask again: 'Are you sure?'

The smile and another gaze to the left reassured me.

Rob's parents Irene and Geoff were, as always, happy to look after Rob for the night and they instructed me to go out and enjoy myself.

I followed their advice; it was a brilliant night. Angela lives an hour from me, in Bedale, but she is so busy with her two young boys and working for an ice-cream business with her husband, Ross, that we don't get together as often as we would like. But she is one of those friends that it doesn't matter how much time has passed since we were last together. As soon as we're in each other's company the conversation and laughter flows.

Angela's friends were fun, too, and the atmosphere at the stadium was amazing. I've never been a drinker but, even sober, we felt giddy enough just singing along and dancing to the songs we once played on a loop in our bedrooms while dreaming about meeting Mark Owen or some boy we might have liked in Year 8.

As Angela said, we danced and laughed like we had not done in years. It was such a special night and I felt rejuvenated driving back to Pontefract.

We had a packed weekend ahead and when I picked up Rob from his parents' house, I was worried about him. He didn't look well but he was emphatic that he wanted to come with me to watch Jackson at his football training, which began at ten-thirty. We had a nice routine every Saturday morning: as soon as we arrived at football, I would zip across and get Rob a coffee, which he loved drinking while watching Jackson run around and play a game with his teammates. But that morning was different. Rob turned his eyes to the right when I offered him his coffee. He didn't want even a sip. This was so unusual for Rob – a man who loved caffeine more than anyone I'd ever known.

I put my hand on his brow. It was hot to the touch. I was sure Rob had a fever but, despite my concern, he refused to allow me to take him home. He wanted to stay and watch Jackson.

By the time we got home Rob was ready for bed. Again, this was so unlike him. He normally wanted to spend as much time as he could with the kids on the weekend. Maybe he'd just had a bad night at his mum's as he'd slept in the reclining chair rather than his own bed. I closed the door softly behind him in the hope he could rest.

We had a big evening ahead as the five of us were due to go to the circus, as we do every year, followed by a meal at Farmer Copleys – which we all love. It has fields where you can pick your own strawberries, a couple of farm dogs (Elfie, a white Jack Russell and Jasper, a black Labrador), a shop, a café and a restaurant. We often go to Farmer Copleys for special occasions but I was sure it would be too much for Rob.

When I woke him in the middle of the afternoon, I fully expected him to say he didn't want to go out. But Rob was determined. His look to the left was emphatic. He wanted to be with us.

The kids were excited and we ended up having a wonderful time at both the circus and Farmer Copleys. The days of Rob ordering something off the menu had long gone and he wasn't interested in the shakes I had packed. I knew he was feeling poorly but Rob kept smiling at the kids.

The thermometer confirmed that Rob had a temperature when we got home. Once I had got him and the children to bed I texted his mum. I didn't want to worry Irene but I explained that Rob had a fever and I needed to drive Macy and Maya to Leeds in the morning. It would be the first dress rehearsal for their drama group Scala's annual *Magic of the Musicals* show the following Friday and Saturday nights. I asked Irene if it would be okay to drop Rob off in the morning – assuming his symptoms were unchanged. Once I got the girls to Leeds I would come back to be with Rob before returning to the rehearsal that afternoon.

After thanking Irene, I didn't shut down my phone; instead I opened up Google and typed three sad words into the search engine: *signs of death*.

I stared at the screen. The first signs that came up all applied to Rob. He was no longer eating, he had a temperature, his breathing was laboured and he was sleeping most of the time.

My next online search was just two words: *child bereavement*.

I knew how important it would be to prepare the children for the death of their dad – but I wished I had spent more time researching bereavement. I wished I had a crystal ball or a simple handbook to tell me what to do and what to say. How would I ensure that Macy, Maya and Jackson continued to have a happy childhood? What long-term effect would Rob's death have on them? Did I need to try and play the role of a dad as well? Was me just being their mum going to be enough for them?

As these questions swirled through me, I was swamped with self-doubt and uncertainty. All I really knew was that I just wanted to protect our children from the inevitable heartache.

After reading a few articles, I felt like I was sinking in quicksand. I hoped desperately that my sixth sense, which had surged through me all evening, was askew.

Rob was still an incredible fighter. He had fought MND with courage and determination for 223 weeks. But he was not done yet. When I woke him as gently as I could that Sunday morning he was alert. There was also a fire in his beautiful blue eyes when I suggested that he miss the trip to Leeds and spend the day at his parents' instead.

'That might be best, darling,' I said softly. 'You're not well.'

Rob turned his gaze to the right in a very firm no.

'Do you really feel up to it?' I asked.

Rob looked to the left with the most adamant stare he could muster.

I cradled him in my arms. 'I'm glad,' I said. 'I would have missed you so much.'

My dad once said that he was worried about trying to pick up Rob because it felt as if his hands might go through skin that felt like thin parchment to the touch. It was different for me. Rob was my husband and I loved holding him. We still made a snug fit as I cuddled him and whispered that we would have a wonderful day with Jackson.

His sisters were so lively and busy, and they made such a team dancing and singing, that Rob and I occasionally worried that Jackson might feel overshadowed. Macy was twelve, Maya was nine and Jackson was five and the girls were much louder and more confident than our little boy, who was less outgoing. Rob worried that Jackson had missed out on having 'a proper dad' from his first birthday onwards, but we all develop at different stages. Jackson was doing well at school and a delight to be around. But, like Rob, I felt we needed to make sure that we gave him special attention.

Jackson helped us plan our day. Once we dropped off the girls at Scala in Leeds we went to the movies. Jackson had chosen *Super Wings* and in more ordinary times Rob would have relished watching an animated movie with our little boy. But, whenever I glanced across in the dark, Rob's eyes were closed.

We then took Jackson swimming and, later that afternoon, once we were home, my parents came over because Leeds United and Southampton were about to meet in the Championship play-off final. My dad, a mad-keen Leeds fan for so many decades, asked Rob if he would like to watch the game. Normally Rob would have been enthusiastic, especially with Leeds having a chance to go up to the Premier League, but he wanted to lie down in bed instead. He might have known from painful experience that Leeds were destined to play terribly that afternoon as they lost 1–0. The dream was over for another year.

The sense grew that we had entered a dark zone, a kind of limbo between life and death. Rob's serious bout of pneumonia the previous summer had prepared me. I mentioned to my mum that I didn't think we had much time left but, otherwise, I kept quiet.

Rob looked better after resting in bed all afternoon. My parents had gone back home and I felt the urge to make it a memorable evening for us as a family. We didn't spend much money going out and we hadn't had a family holiday in years. So Rob had needed little persuading when I'd suggested that, for once, we splash out and pay for a cinema room to be built in the house. I knew how much Rob loved the movies and the chance to watch films on a big screen at home was irresistible.

The chairs had yet to arrive but the cinema room itself was completed. Rob had not been well enough to be taken upstairs but the kids were so excited about seeing *Wonka* that I asked Rob if he felt well enough for me to lift him up so that he could join us.

The familiar smile and movement of his eyes to the left had the kids cheering.

I knew my mum and dad would have scolded me for doing it on my own but I eased Rob out of his chair and, carefully, lifted him from behind. It was always surprising how much heavier he was to carry than expected. I climbed the stairs steadily, taking each one slowly as the thought of what might happen to Rob if I fell was terrifying. Throughout 2020 and much of 2021 I had made this sad journey every night as I carried Rob up to bed, but for the previous two years he had lived in a room downstairs. So I felt out of practice and a little tentative as we approached the top of the staircase.

But then we were on the landing and I soon had Rob safely in a chair in the cinema room. His smile was wide as he looked around. The kids jumped up and down excitedly, talking over each other in their haste to tell Rob all about the room, the movie and the soft drinks and popcorn I had lined up for them.

They only quietened down when I dimmed the lights and the opening scenes of *Wonka* spooled across the screen. The room was lit by a blue hue that cast beautiful shadows across the faces of Rob and the children. I let slip a sigh of relief. It had all been worth it. They were lost in the deliciously chocolatey world of Willy Wonka.

I knew Rob was too unwell to be able to watch another film ever again. But the last movie of his life, at home with me and the kids in our new cinema room, felt as special as it was moving.

The next day was a Bank Holiday Monday, and we kept up the pace. Rob was again insistent that he would join Jackson and me in Leeds after we took the girls back to Scala. We went to Roundhay Park, Tropical World and then Leeds Bradford Airport where, from the car park, we watched the planes taking off. Jackson was thrilled and Rob smiled at me before declining my offer of a shake. He had eaten nothing all day.

It mattered more to Rob that we had made some beautiful memories for Jackson in those two days together. He knew, better than me, that time was short.

Before I went into work at the hospital on the morning of Tuesday 28 May, and while I was making breakfast for the kids, I heard Rob coughing in his room. He would usually be asleep until I woke him and prepared him for a day with his parents every Tuesday. I was immediately worried and went to see Rob.

We used our eye-moving method and Rob indicated he was feeling better again and that he was happy for me to go to work. It was typical Rob.

Irene arrived on time, as always, to look after Rob. We all

kissed him goodbye, and hugged him close, not knowing then that he would never see our house again.

I had a really busy time at work and, as my phone signal is hopeless at the hospital, I was not in contact with anyone from home all day. It was only when I walked to the car around 5pm that I picked up a message from Rob's sister Claire. She said I was not to panic but they'd had the doctor out and he'd advised them to take Rob to Pinderfields Hospital in Wakefield.

I rang Claire, my heart racing and my head whirring. They were still in A&E and Claire told me they thought Rob had a chest infection and he was about to be admitted. I went into practical mode. 'Right,' I said, 'I'll pick up the girls and, after I get them home, I'll come straight to the hospital.'

I did my best to shield the children from Rob's condition but I could be honest with my mum. 'He won't come home this time,' I said softly.

I drove to Pinderfields in a daze. When I arrived they had moved Rob to a respiratory ward. Room 1, Gate 27.

I tried to stay strong when I finally saw Rob, an oxygen mask strapped to his face. I kissed him and stroked his arm while saying hello to Claire and Irene.

A senior nurse reassured me that everything was being done for Rob. He was comfortable and, once the consultants had finished conferring, they would discuss a plan of care with us.

But the nursing sister also said it was important that we protected Rob from public attention. She reminded us he was a high-profile case as Rob was so well known. Even though the media had treated us with great respect we needed to set up a password to keep out everyone but family members and close friends.

The nurse asked if there was a particular password we wanted to use.

Before anyone else could answer I said the word that described Rob best: *Hero*.

10

Look to the Left to Say Goodbye

Wednesday 29 May 2024, Pinderfields Hospital,
Wakefield

Rob has been diagnosed with aspiration pneumonia, which is an infection of the lungs caused by food, liquid or saliva being breathed into the airways. It usually affects elderly people but it can also occur when a younger patient has difficulties swallowing. Days have passed since Rob drank one of the prescribed shakes, but his lungs have probably been contaminated by inhaling bacterial-rich fluids from his stomach or the back of his throat. It has become a struggle for him to breathe.

But by Wednesday afternoon, almost twenty-four hours after his admission to Pinderfields, the antibiotics have begun to make a difference. His white blood cell count has come down and they've taken him off the low-flow oxygen machine. These positive signs lift me but Dr Lowe, the palliative care consultant, explains that sometimes an end-of-life patient will rally briefly. It's her way of reminding me that it is important not to cling to false hope. Rob is still extremely poorly.

I protect the children as much as I can, without making any

false promises. But Macy, being the eldest, is worried. 'Mum,' she says, 'maybe we shouldn't do the Scala show?'

We are just three nights away from their big night and so I ask Rob if the girls should withdraw from the production so that they can be with us in hospital.

Rob is adamant as he moves his eyes to the right. It's a clear 'no', but I ask him again in a different way: 'Are you really sure you want them to do the show?'

His eyes move in the opposite direction, to the left, to tell me 'yes'.

He knows how much musical theatre means to the girls. *Magic of the Musicals* is to be held at the Yeadon Town Hall Theatre, on the edge of Leeds, and Macy, Maya and their friends at Scala have been working hard for months on their songs and dance routines. Rob, Jackson and I have tickets for the Saturday night and I've already asked the main consultant at Pinderfields if he thinks there's a chance we will be able to attend. He looks very doubtful but said we will see how Rob responds after another day of antibiotics. But, deep down, we know that Rob will not make it. Yeadon is an hour's drive away and it will also be too much for him to sit through a long production.

But I share Rob's conviction that the girls should perform. They love being on stage, and they will be at the hospital the rest of the time. While Jackson is happy staying with my parents, the hospital has agreed that Macy and Maya can sleep every night in the room they have arranged for me at Pinderfields. The girls take the two reclining chairs which turn into makeshift beds, while I'm happy dozing in an ordinary chair alongside them or Rob.

Macy and Maya are wonderful company; despite the sadness, they keep me amused and entertained. And, whenever I look low, they instinctively know how to cheer me up. Even though I insist that I am 'fine', which is the word I use more than any other when trying to deflect attention from my sadness, they cuddle me and tell me that I am the best mum in the world and that they love me.

They also make me laugh because they do not spare me when I admit they did not inherit their performing talents from their old mum. When asked if I am better at singing, dancing or football, Maya answers decisively: 'She can't dance and she can't sing for toffee. So it has to be football.'

Her big sister makes sure to keep even that in check. Macy says my football prowess remains at 'tot level' since I had last kicked a ball back and forth to Jackson when he first started training on Saturday mornings as a very little boy. But even my tiny tot football is less embarrassing to the girls than my hopeless dancing and terrible singing.

I've provided many embarrassing mum moments but, for Maya, the most excruciating was when, walking her to school one day, I began an impromptu dance exercise routine. Nine-year-old Maya quickly walked ahead of me while saying, in a voice as exasperated as it was sensible, 'I don't know this woman . . . I definitely don't know this woman.'

But they are generous and loving. When asked to compare me to an animal or a bird, Maya says I remind her of a lioness because I am 'fearless'. Macy turns to Greek mythology when she chooses a phoenix, because it is a bird that rises from the ashes. I resemble a phoenix because I am 'brave'.

It does not sound quite as flattering when, asked to pick a character in a book or a musical that reminds them of me, they initially settle on Humpty Dumpty. I laugh but they point out that it is a serious compliment because, while all the king's horses and all the king's men couldn't put Humpty together again after his great fall, I am very good at getting up and patching myself together again. Macy then compares me to Jenna in the musical *Waitress* because 'she goes through loads of hard times but in the end she makes it all work and powers through because she's such a superhero'.

I certainly don't feel brave, fearless or heroic in Pinderfields. There are times when I feel lost, desolate and a little scared as I gaze at Rob. I try to let him sleep and rest as much as he can. When the girls are away rehearsing, I spend a lot of time with Jackson, watching videos together or playing games, and so Geoff and Irene and my parents often sit with Rob. He is incapable of much communication and the four of them pass the time chatting to each other.

While discussing how special the nursing staff at Pinder-fields are they begin reminiscing about the days when you could expect such expert care and efficiency as a matter of routine. They all remember how they could just turn up at the local GP practice in Castleford and wait in a small queue for a helpful appointment that same morning or afternoon. It is no longer possible to do this anywhere in the country. They are not moaning – just acknowledging how much the health system, and life itself, has changed.

Thursday 30 May 2024, Pinderfields Hospital, Wakefield

I sit in a corner of Rob's room with Jackson. A little DVD player balances on my lap as we watch *Ghostbusters* together. Irene and my Auntie Sue and Uncle Roy are at Rob's bedside. Geoff has gone down to the café to get some Eccles cakes. The room is calm and quiet, apart from the soft burble of sound from the DVD player. It is nearly lunchtime but Jackson is lost in the movie, while I settle into the peace of the moment.

Then, with a brutal jolt, everything changes.

Rob is suddenly struggling to breathe. He is fighting desperately for oxygen and his breathing is high and jagged. One of the machines makes a beeping sound.

Rising from my chair in distress, I call out to the nurses. They arrive quickly and there is an intense flurry of activity. I turn away to make sure Jackson is all right. There are more beeps and cries and, while I try to reassure Jackson, the room fills with people. Specialists, consultants and nurses gather around Rob.

I hear snatches of fraught conversation and pointed instruction. I know enough to understand that Rob's sats have dropped horribly. These numbers confirm how much oxygen is currently flowing through the blood; a healthy adult will have an oxygen saturation level between 95 and 100 per cent. From the agitation in the medical voices around me I can tell

Rob's sats have plummeted to a deeply concerning low. Anything below 90 per cent is considered as hypoxemia and I fear that Rob has entered this red zone.

We are surrounded by highly trained professionals, but for a few terrifying moments, panic seems to fill the room. It feels like I am watching a big, messy ER scene in an upsetting movie.

One of the consultants looks up and sees me. I ask if we should take Jackson out of the room. 'Yes,' she says firmly. I turn to my aunt and uncle and they are already reaching out to Jackson. They know we need to get my little boy away from here, to a safe place where no one is talking urgently or scarily. I ask Sue and Roy to take Jackson to my mum and dad.

Irene is visibly upset and soon I'll try and comfort her. But, first, I turn back to the monitor. My eyes fix on the screen, yearning for Rob's oxygen saturation levels and heart rate to start rising again. I whisper words in my head: *Come on, Rob. Please, come on. Just get through this. We're all here, rooting for you . . .*

The room calms eventually. Rob is on oxygen again, his face covered by a mask while the ventilator keeps him alive. It is a scary sight but all my years in healthcare steel me. I remain in charge of my emotions until the consultant comes over. She tells me what I already know about the sat levels and then adds another gentle, but devastating, sentence: 'I think you should get your children.'

I know what this means. We are going to lose Rob. Macy, Maya and little Jackson are going to lose their dad.

I look into her face, searching for fleeting reassurance, but she has to be clear and honest. It takes a moment and then I hear myself say: 'I don't think I want them to see their dad like this.'

The consultant gives a little nod to show that she understands. But she won't allow herself, or me, to waver. 'He's critical,' she says.

I know she's right and so I leave the room. I walk down the corridor and find a place where I can make some calls. It's half term and so I phone Scala first and, when a woman answers, I explain that Rob is very poorly. Will she talk to Macy and Maya and hear if they want to come back to see their dad? But I stress that, if they don't want to, then I'm happy for them to stay at Scala.

I phone my mum next and ask her to bring Jackson back as soon as Sue arrives with him. 'Come as quick as you can, Mum,' I say. 'I don't think we've got long.'

The lady at Scala soon calls me to say the girls want to see their dad.

'How are they?' I ask.

'They're upset,' she says, 'but they both want to be with you.'

It helps calm me, knowing that the children are on their way and that I can now be with Rob. I won't ever forgive myself if I am missing when he slips away.

I take my familiar place at his bedside, with Geoff and Irene sitting opposite. We talk a little and then, in the silence, I bolster myself by reverting to a medical routine. My fingers rest lightly on Rob's wrist as I check his pulse. All the time, with my voice a silent echo in my head, I urge him on. *Keep fighting. Come on, Rob.*

Macy, Maya and Jackson are back with me. We're all upset but at least we are together. My parents and Rob's parents and sisters are also with us. We are shown into a family room where the consultant will talk to all of us. She has just told me that I have done the right thing, bringing the children back, and that she will explain everything with their needs uppermost in mind. I trust her and I hug the children before saying the doctor will now talk about their daddy. She will help us to understand everything.

Jackson looks frightened and so I kiss him gently. I do the same to both Maya and Macy.

The consultant is wonderful. She is as clear as she is compassionate. She explains, with delicate tenderness, that we will soon go into the room to see their daddy. It is time to say goodbye and, while it is very sad, it is important we remember that he won't suffer any more pain. Her tone is comforting and the children are not distraught. They are calm and attentive and I can tell that even little Jackson is listening closely. The consultant tells them not to be worried when they walk into the room. There will be lights and noises, machines and masks, bags and tubes, but everything is helping their dad.

She talks for twenty minutes and offers an incredibly balanced mix of truth and care. We all feel better having listened to her. The consultant eventually says: 'Are there any questions?'

Macy looks up, as beautiful as she is composed, and asks a simple question: 'Can I go and see my daddy, please?'

The consultant smiles. 'Of course you can.'

My mum speaks next. 'Lindsey, you just go with the children.'

It's typical of Mum, finding a way for us to have time alone with Rob, but Jackson has a different idea. 'I want Grandpa,' he says, looking up at my dad. 'Grandpa, you've got to come.'

I smile at my little boy and my dad, and then at everyone else. 'Let's all go in together,' I suggest.

Jackson slips his tiny hand into my father's hand and leads the way. 'Come on, Grandpa,' he says reassuringly, 'you don't need to be scared. Remember what the lady said – all them lights and noises and tubes are helping Daddy.'

Macy, however, has begun to cry heartfelt tears. She lies down on the bed and holds Rob tight.

Rob opens his eyes. I think he hears Macy saying how much she loves him. Maya is next. She copies her big sister and stretches out on the bed. 'I love you, Daddy,' she says, while crying. 'You're the best daddy in the world.'

I allow the girls to have this moment but it feels as if my heart might break. But then I hear Jackson. He is still looking after my dad.

'It's all right, Grandpa,' Jackson says. 'Don't be sad. The flashing lights are helping Daddy.'

Macy turns to my mum. 'Bring Jackson here, Nanna. He needs to come and kiss Daddy goodbye. He needs to tell him he loves him.'

My mum picks up Jackson and carries him to the bed. As

she walks she sees two nurses in the corner of the room. Tears stream down their faces.

Jackson looks at Rob and climbs across the bed. His tiny arms stretch out to clutch the withered frame of his dad. He echoes his sisters as he says: 'I love you, Daddy. You're the best daddy. Goodbye, Daddy.'

He then turns to look at my dad. 'Can we go now, Grandpa?' he asks. 'Can we go?'

I bring all the children close to me. I tell them it's time to leave the room and give everyone else a chance to say goodbye. They seem calm as I lead them out and I feel we have done the right thing. We have not told them that Rob is going to sleep or to heaven. We have told them the truth and they have accepted it. Their tears are raw and natural. They understand what's happening and I am sure this will help them in the weeks, months and years ahead.

When my mum and dad come out to join us, they have also said their goodbyes to Rob. They kept it simple. My mum said: 'Goodbye, Rob. It'll be all right. We'll look after them.'

My dad also offered reassurance as he squeezed Rob's hand. 'They'll be fine, Rob. We'll make sure of it.'

I wait until everyone has had their turn and I go in alone to see Rob. His eyes are closed. I tell Rob how much I love him, and I thank him for everything he has given me, and us as a family. We have had a wonderful life together and I want him to know there is no need to worry. I will look after Macy, Maya and Jackson. I will make sure I keep bringing them up in the way we've always wanted. They will be polite and kind and I will strive to give them every opportunity they deserve. I will do Rob proud, and I will never let him, or the children, down.

I don't say goodbye yet because I still can't quite believe it.

After the shock and the tears I was still not entirely surprised when, late that afternoon, Rob rallied. He was Rob Burrow, after all, and so he fought back.

His skin was still grey, with his face covered in a mask, but he looked a little better. I didn't want to say anything as I was not sure if I had imagined that slight improvement.

It was only when a different consultant came in that I began to believe we would not lose Rob quite yet. She told me that she had better news.

Two sets of blood results had been assessed and she said that Rob had come through something called Lazarus syndrome. I didn't understand at first but, then, it sounded miraculous. Lazarus syndrome occurs when blood circulation returns spontaneously after the heart stops beating. The blood tests told us that, just after lunchtime, Rob had basically come back from the dead.

Rob, I thought, *what a man you are . . .*

If I had not seen him fighting so hard against MND for the previous four and a half years I would not have believed it was possible. But Rob was back with us.

'His bloods are showing signs of recovery,' the consultant said. 'We're going to move him to the respiratory ward.'

I knew that there would be no lasting miracle. Rob would

not come home but, still, gratitude surged through me. We had him with us for a little while longer.

Kevin Sinfield had been on edge since Tuesday evening. He was one of the few people I had messaged when Rob was hospitalised and, typical of Kev, he was all set to immediately leave the England rugby union training camp at Pennyhill Park in Bagshot, Surrey, and drive the 205 miles to reach Pinderfields. England, for whom Kev was a key member of their coaching staff, were preparing for a summer tour of Japan and New Zealand but they understood how much he cared about Rob. Geoff and I persuaded Kev that we would update him and, until we had more definite news, it made sense for him to keep working in Surrey.

When Rob's condition rapidly deteriorated I again made contact with Kev after lunchtime on Thursday; he stressed that he would reach Wakefield early that evening. After picking up his wife, Jayne, from their home near Oldham, Kev arrived at Pinderfields still wearing his England training kit. Although we have known Jayne for years, she wanted Kev to see Rob on his own as their time together would be so precious.

Irene and Joanne were at Rob's bedside when Kev walked into the hushed room. Kev is such a respectful and serious person but he instantly found the right tone. 'So what's going on here?' he joked with Rob. 'I've rushed all this way to see you and you're lying there grinning at me. What are you up to now?'

Rob kept smiling. He and Kev had shared so much that the

bonds ran deep. And then, of course, something truly beautiful had unfolded between them over the past four and a half years. Kev had pushed himself to the brink of intense suffering with his 24-hour runs and ultra-marathons to raise millions for MND in honour of the smallest Rhino. Rob, meanwhile, defied his own silent suffering to spread awareness of MND while showing us all how to live.

In a deeply moving moment, Kev bent down to cuddle him. But he knew that Rob would not wish him to be sentimental or miserable. So Kev started to joke again as he stepped back to look at Rob, who still had an oxygen mask strapped to his face.

'I can't believe it,' Kev said. 'You've got a new moustache again?'

Beneath the filmy covering of the mask, Kev could see the faint moustache that had begun to grow across Rob's upper lip. 'At least it goes with the dyed hair up top.'

Kev kept on ribbing him and brought up the amusing fact that Rob, as a young player in Super League, used to top up his fake winter tan on a sunbed. 'It matched the highlights in your hair,' Kev remembered. He paused and then, looking down fondly at his friend, he added: 'Rob, you're still the only player I ever knew who brought hair straighteners with him to a game.'

Rob wheezed with laughter because it was all true. And so the next forty-five minutes passed easily. Even when the mickey-taking stopped, Rob kept smiling as Kev chatted away.

But beneath the gentle humour and attempt to include Rob in all they discussed, Kev knew that the last goodbye could not be held back for much longer. Rob looked exhausted and, after hugging Irene and Joanne, Kev turned to him one final time. They had been through heartache and glory, sorrow and joy – and so the look between these two warriors went beyond language.

Kev leaned down to kiss Rob on his damp forehead. 'Love you, pal,' he said softly.

And then, slowly, Kev turned away. He knew he would never see Rob again.

It was time to message Barrie McDermott. Ever since he was a young player breaking into the Leeds Rhinos squad, Rob had looked up to Barrie, a man who combines great strength with wry kindness. They had forged a deep friendship.

Barrie had always bolstered Rob, and he also put up with his relentless taunting and teasing. He even forgave Rob his strange and devilish antics – from weeing on furious players in the shower after training to moving their cars so far away they thought they had been stolen – and never thought about throttling him.

Barrie traded insults and wisecracks with Rob but, more importantly, he took care of my husband. When Rob was hurting, he would turn to Barrie. Whether it was his disappointment at losing his place in the starting thirteen, or struggling in the more complicated world of coaching, Rob always turned to

Barrie for advice and sustenance. Barrie was his great friend and mentor. And once MND brought darkness into our lives, only Barrie could still make Rob laugh so much that he began farting uncontrollably.

I knew how important it was to stay in touch with Barrie, even when I felt so frayed and sad.

Sitting at Rob's bedside I wrote my text late that Thursday night:

> Hi Barrie. I wanted to let you know Rob became acutely unwell at lunchtime today. He was struggling to breathe and his oxygen saturations were extremely low. The consultant advised me to get the kids. They've put him on some antibiotics and a ventilator and he is now much more stable but still very poorly. They've moved him to the respiratory ward. I'll keep you updated. Lindsey xx.

Barrie picked up my message just after 6am the next morning. I was already awake when my phone pinged with his reply. *Thanks Lindsey. Thinking of you. Would it be okay to come and see him today?*

Of course, I replied. *I'm at the hospital with the girls and Rob's mum. The password to get in is Hero. He's on Gate 27, Room 1.*

Barrie arrived early that morning, just before 8am. When she saw him, Irene punched the air with a sudden burst of happiness. Geoff just beamed. It meant so much because, like me, they knew how much Rob loved Barrie. He kissed Irene and

233

me, shook Geoff's hand, said hello to the girls, and then started chatting to Rob.

The oxygen mask was still strapped tightly to Rob's face but his eyes were open and, from the way they crinkled, we could tell he was smiling. It was another sign of how he came to life in the company of a beloved teammate from the Rhinos. I felt it was only right to give them some privacy; it was also time to get the girls their breakfast at the hospital café.

I heard later that, while chatting to Irene and Geoff, Barrie kept involving Rob. It was a good visit and at the end, Barrie did what he was always did. The great big prop forward kissed Rob on his forehead – just as Kev had done twelve hours earlier. Barrie told Rob he loved him and that he would see him later.

Barrie believed it, too. Unlike Kev, who knew that we were down to the last day or two, Barrie thought that Rob would rally again. He had marvelled at Rob's ability to rise up against all the odds for the twenty-five years they had known each other. The last few months and weeks had also shown Barrie how deep Rob would dig to fight for every last breath. As he reached his car Barrie thought: *Rob will pick up, he'll get better and he'll be home before we know it. I'll see my little pal soon.*

After I texted Barrie to say how much it had meant to us to see him, he replied:

Thank you for letting me visit. Hopefully it helped pass an hour for you all. Always there for you and Rob. He is a fighter, Lindsey. I'm in constant awe of him. How is he?

There was no point worrying Barrie and so I wrote:

Hi, Baz, he's settled. His obs have been stable all day. He's such a fighter. I couldn't be more proud of him if I tried.

Rob had, once more, used his eyes to communicate his desire for the girls to keep going with the show. He wanted me with him most of the day but we had agreed that, if he was well enough, I would be backstage that Friday evening at their first performance. I wanted to be with Rob but I also felt the girls needed me. So I drove them to Leeds that morning as Maya had been complaining of a tummy ache. I knew she was upset so I calmed her down and managed to see snippets of the rehearsal. Macy and Maya were stunning on stage and I think only a few people knew that their dad was critically ill.

The girls were hopeful I would be back to help them get ready that evening, as long as I could leave Rob, and so I felt better as I returned to Pinderfields.

Rob slept most of the day but late that afternoon he encouraged me to return to Leeds. His parents and sisters were with him and Jackson was safe at my mum and dad's house. It felt important to look after Maya, in case of another wobble, and to support Macy too. So back to Leeds I went, feeling torn all over again at leaving Rob.

But it eventually turned out to be a special evening. Although I didn't see the show as I was backstage, I could help the girls and their friends with all the changes of costume and act as a chaperone. Macy and Maya didn't really need me in the end, as they were so caught up in the production, which received a rapturous reception.

The clapping and cheering were still ringing in our ears when we reached the hospital at around ten that night. Rob was asleep in his room and the nursing staff reassured me that he was stable.

In the relatives' room, I tucked Macy and Maya up in bed. I settled down in my chair and, despite the discomfort, drifted off to sleep soon after them.

Saturday 1 June 2024, Pinderfields Hospital, Wakefield

As pale sunshine spreads across Wakefield, Rob cannot hide his agony. When I ask him if the pain is really bad his eyes shift to the left in a mute reply of 'yes'. I reassure him that we will get help. I go in search of a nurse who tracks down the consult-ant. She says that the pain could be caused by the pneumonia or chest problems associated with his heart.

Rob's eyes are sunk deep into their sockets but I see them flicker to the right when the consultant suggests that we take an ECG to check his heart.

'Do you want the ECG now?' I ask.

Rob's eyes turn to the right again in a defiant no. 'Maybe later?' I suggest.

The same rightwards glance repeats Rob's answer – as it does when the doctor asks if she can call the respiratory physio to help his breathing with some gentle massage.

But Rob doesn't want to see a physio. The consultant leaves quietly and I sit on my own in the room with Rob.

The morning passes and the pattern is set. Rob keeps moving his eyes to the right, saying no to everything. He won't use his nasal spray. He won't take any more medication. He doesn't even want a small drink.

I know what he is telling me. He's had enough. It's time.

I go in search of the consultant. I trust her and I need to tell her that I think Rob is giving in.

She nods and says that she is pleased I've come to see her. She had been preparing to find me to have this difficult conversation. She explains that they don't expect that Rob will ever be able to come off the ventilator. It is her way of telling me we've reached the end.

I feel the same. If they reduce the pressure on the ventilator and allow Rob's breathing to slow, while ensuring he is comfortable and out of pain, it will be the most humane step towards ending his suffering. But I need to know how Rob truly feels. This needs to be his decision.

I return to the room where I am soon joined by a senior palliative care nurse.

'Rob,' I say, 'I know you're really tired.'

His eyes fix on me in an unblinking stare. He hardly looks like Rob anymore. His trauma now seems unbearable and so I have to ask this question.

'Rob,' I say, as gently as I can, 'have you had enough?'

There is silence in the room. And then, clearly and unmistakably, Rob looks to the left.

I want to cry but I need to make sure. 'Rob,' I say, 'if you look to the left you're telling me you've had enough. Is that what you really mean?'

Rob looks to the left again. He has no voice, but I still hear him.

I am heartbroken but this is not about me, or anyone else. This is about Rob. I want him to feel he can let go now. I want him to know that he can stop fighting and stop suffering. I want him to be released from the pain of MND, even if it means we have to say goodbye to him. We can let him go peacefully, knowing how much we love him.

But I feel torn apart. I have been an advocate for Rob's positivity and sheer fight for so long and now it feels as if I am the one telling him to give up.

'Rob,' I say, my voice cracking. 'Please tell me that I've not put pressure on you. I hope that's not how you feel?'

Rob finds it within himself to say 'no' by looking to the right.

I know he would say more, and do more, if he could. But he can't and so I hold him in my arms for a long time.

When Rob eventually falls back to sleep I have to leave the room otherwise I might howl. The palliative care nurse suggests we have a chat in a small office. She is incredible because I am devastated and have already begun torturing myself.

The door has barely shut behind us before I say the guilt-stricken words: 'Maybe I forced him to make that decision.' I begin to cry. 'Maybe I've talked him into it? Should I have just said: "Do you want to keep fighting?"'

The nurse reassures me over and over again. 'You were brilliant,' she says kindly, 'and you haven't pressurised him. Rob isn't going to get better so, I promise you, this is the right thing.'

Geoff is distraught when he hears the news from the consultant. He thinks the hospital have given up on Rob. Geoff still believes we just need to get Rob breathing without the machine and then we will help him get better. My heart aches for Geoff as I can see the strain on his face. Irene has already told me how upset he has been at home. It took them a long time to reach the hospital late this morning.

Geoff has always refused to give in to the harsh realities of MND. Whenever we told him that it was incurable Geoff would reach for a paper he had just found on the internet, which showed that great strides were being made in America. Trials were being held and encouraging results had been returned. We just needed to believe a little harder and maybe Rob could live until a cure was fully developed.

Rob and I understood that his dad was just trying to find hope amid the wreckage. So we listened patiently, and loved Geoff for his defiance and optimism.

But now is the time for truth. Rob doesn't want to go on any longer. And my truth is that I want Rob to be at peace. I also don't want the children to see him like this much longer. I want him to be comfortable, surrounded by all of us, while death comes as a merciful relief to Rob.

The consultant talks to Geoff, Irene and Joanne. Geoff is very distressed as he thinks that they will just turn the machine off. The consultant explains that this is not the case. They will gradually lessen the intensity of the ventilator so Rob, with the help of morphine's pain relief, can slip away. But Geoff is still adamant that Rob should fight on.

Joanne comes to see me. She tells me that we are doing the right thing. 'My dad's upset,' she says, 'but I've had to be quite firm with him. I've said: "Dad, they're not putting pressure on Rob. The pneumonia's got worse and we have to think of Rob and what he wants now."'

The consensus might not be quite unanimous yet. But Irene, Joanne, Claire, the hospital and I all agree with Rob. We know that he has had enough.

Saturday evening is strangely tranquil. The children are at the show in Yeadon with my parents, after Rob had again moved his eyes to the left to indicate that he wanted the girls to per-form, and I am with Irene, Claire and Joanne. We are in Rob's room and we have placed the little DVD player on a stand so that he can watch our wedding video with us. Most of the time we just chat but we also really watch and laugh, and cry too, when we reach our first dance at the wedding.

We tease Rob about how hard he worked to look good that night – and it worked. He looks great, moving and dancing fluidly across the screen on that beautiful day on 30 December 2006. Seventeen and a half years have passed since then and, as I hold his hand, I think how lucky I've been. I lived that song with Rob and I've really had the time of my life. We've had the time of our lives.

When the video ends, and beyond the hum of the ventilator,

the room is hushed. I know this is not about me. My thoughts are now with the children. We are about to face a traumatic twenty-four hours, and life beyond that is streaked with uncertainty. What's going to happen? How am I going to support them? I feel the weight of responsibility but I am calm too. Rob's eyes are closed but I tell him I will find a way. I promise to look after them and to make sure that they are happy and fulfilled – and that they will never forget how extraordinary he has always been.

Geoff, who was so stressed that he was taken home, is in contact as *Britain's Got Talent* spools across the television screen in a corner of Rob's room. I have been worried about Geoff. I know how much has been taken from him – especially these last few days. I know that Geoff would never think I've abandoned Rob but, still, it's a relief when he sends Irene a lovely message on our family WhatsApp group. *I am fine, darling*, he begins as he outlines a possible scenario for me to share with Rob. Geoff suggests that we slowly try to reduce Rob's dependence on the machine. We could do this in short bursts and see what transpires. Geoff signs off by saying: *Tell Rob: we can, we will. I can, I will. That's what we said when Rob got diagnosed and I hope Rob agrees.*

I feel enormous empathy for Geoff. I can only imagine how hard it must be to lose your son or daughter.

Rob is awake now and the next forty minutes pass in a blur of our shared pride and love for the children. I asked Louise, the Scala choreographer, if she could send us videos of Macy and Maya's solos and central performances from *Magic of the Musicals*. This year they are doing extracts from *Annie*, *School of Rock*, *Mamma Mia*, *13* and other productions, as well as – almost in honour of Rob the superfan – a tribute to Michael Jackson.

The highlights reel of the Burrow girls has me cheering and welling up, along with Irene, Claire and Joanne, while Rob grins at the screen. I can see again how he idolises our three beauties. We all feel like bursting with pride when Maya sings a big solo – 'Castle on a Cloud' from *Les Miserables*. Macy is drowning in a big American football top with the number 12 on it, but she also nails her solo from the musical *13*. Maya will tell me later how nervous she was 'in the wings', sounding like a real musical theatre pro, and worrying, 'What happens if I mess up?'

But rather than messing up both girls get standing ovations and none of us have any idea that they were also concerned about losing their microphones taped to their back pockets while they did cartwheels across the stage.

Their sunshine fills our hospital room. I smile so much, at the screen and at Rob, but my heart also aches. I know that this will be the last of the children's milestones he will ever see. But it feels special to share one last burst of magic.

It is harder for my parents as I messaged my mum in the interval. *Please bring them straight back after the show, Mum*, I text. It's so important that Macy, Maya and Jackson have as much time as possible on their last night with their dad.

*

During the Scala interval my dad had taken Jackson to the toilet. Little Jackson had run ahead and a woman had shouted out: 'He's the spitting image of his father.' My dad just grinned as he raced after Jackson.

That same exuberance flowed through Macy and Maya. They were excited to be reunited with Jackson and they were thrilled with the success of the show. They filled the car journey to Wakefield with songs from the production, only breaking off to cheer, with Jackson, when my dad parked outside a Dominos close to the hospital.

The kids were all starving and they skipped around the little takeaway after choosing their pizzas. They soon made the short walk to Pinderfields and chatted to the patients from the hospital who had slipped outside for a Saturday-night cigarette.

'Those pizzas look tasty,' one old patient said as he saw the giant boxes the kids were carrying.

'You can't have any,' Maya said with a laugh while Macy shouted out a cheerful 'Sorry!'

I was waiting for them in reception and, seeing the riot of colour and hearing their laughter, I stepped outside to meet them. The children came running to me, shouting 'Mummy, Mummy!' I stretched my arms wide to hug them close. Their own arms were too full of pizza boxes to hug me back, but they nuzzled into me.

After I spoke briefly to my parents, and they saw that I had been crying, my mum and dad watched the four of us turn back to the hospital. They both said later they would never forget the silhouette Maya, Macy, Jackson and I made against the glass doors in a haunting, if beautiful, image. The children did not know what awaited them once those glass doors opened.

We still found a way to keep sadness at bay that last unforgettable night in Room 1, Gate 27. As soon as the kids were at Rob's bedside they couldn't help themselves. They talked and laughed, gobbled up pizza and watched videos from the show again and again.

The nurses had brought them ink pads which you normally use to make prints of a newborn baby's tiny hands and feet. The children took great care as they painted Rob's fragile fingers. He was awake but drowsy as he watched them make prints for their memory books. Macy made a little tree out of his fingerprints. The nurses had also given them tiny knitted hearts and bears which the kids used to surround Rob's tree.

Rob's fingers were painted bright red, yellow and green as he watched Macy, Maya and Jackson have fun. In the last photograph I ever took of Rob he is smiling, surrounded by love and his three children.

Midnight came and went and I allowed Macy to watch *Britain's Got Talent* on catch-up. Maya, still wearing her Scala hoodie and with her hair still done up from the show, snuggled against me. Jackson climbed on to Rob's bed. It felt beautiful to be all together as a family, with Irene, Claire and Joanne in the room too.

At around 2am, Joanne and I settled the kids down in the relatives' room. Joanne said she would stay with them so that I could be with Rob.

Before I switched off their light, Macy said softly to me so the others would not hear: 'I'm sad, Mum. Daddy won't ever see me in a Scala show again. He was my number one fan.'

I looked at my gorgeous twelve-year-old girl and smiled. 'Well,' I said, 'can I be your number one fan now?'

Macy nodded and hugged me tight.

It was peaceful as Irene, Claire and I sat through the early hours together with the man who was, in turn, a son, a brother, and, for me, my husband and the love of my life. Sometimes we spoke but, more often, we just sat quietly with our own thoughts, and our beloved Rob.

Sunday 2 June 2024, Pinderfields Hospital, Wakefield

The children and I are led into a room. The palliative care consultant is waiting for us and I know what she is about to say. She tells them that their dad has become increasingly unwell and that she is going to give him medicine to stop him hurting all over. And then, she says: 'After a while we are going to turn the machine off.'

The children understand. They know the end has come. And they want to see Rob.

We're all crying. Macy and Maya echo each other as they say 'Daddy, I love you so much' and 'We love you, Daddy.' It's really hard and I try my utmost to help them. The nurses talk to the children and they've brought them bags of Haribo and Calippo ice lollies. But it's important too that Macy, Maya and Jackson understand that their dad is being looked after so well.

The consultant explains that they have given Rob a dose of morphine, which will take away all his pain. Twenty minutes later they return discreetly and switch off the ventilator and all the monitors around Rob's bed. They remove his mask and even make him look comfortable.

The children are not frightened as they talk to me. I don't know what I had been expecting. Perhaps that, after twenty minutes or even an hour, there would be a dramatic deathbed scene as Rob opened his eyes before he took one last breath.

Instead, he looks peaceful, his eyes closed, and his breathing slow yet steady.

We are also all remarkably steady. The kids watch videos and play with my phone. Joanne falls asleep in my chair and we laugh as Maya takes photos of her snoring softly.

Around lunchtime they give Rob another dose of morphine. My eyes fix on Rob's chest, watching it rise and fall slowly. The children share their sweets with Geoff, Irene, Claire and Joanne. The room is full of love.

It's just after 2pm when I notice that Rob's chest is no longer moving. He looks as serene as he is still.

I turn to the nurse. 'Has he passed?' I ask.

'Yes,' she says.

I lean over to kiss Rob goodbye and then I turn to the children and open my arms. They fill me up as I hold them close.

When they look at their dad, they all cry but they also do something beautiful. They open Rob's hands. His fingers are still painted red and yellow and green and then, telling him how much they love him, they take turns to pour the little knitted hearts from the night before on to his upturned palms. When they close his hands around their hearts it feels complete.

We will carry Rob, their dad, with us for ever.

The four of us are home now. I remember how, earlier in the week, Macy said to me: 'Mummy, do you promise you'll be honest with us and tell us what's happening with Daddy?'

It was a serious and important question and I replied in a similar tone: 'I promise you, hand on my heart, I will tell you everything.'

I feel now that I have kept my promise.

But I also spare the children when my parents come to see me soon after we return from the hospital. I break down in the kitchen with my mum and dad and weep helplessly.

I then compose myself and Maya comes and finds me. She wants to be with me and I ask if she can help me prepare tea for her, Macy and Jackson. Little Maya nods. The kids have not eaten since breakfast, apart from their ice lollies and Haribo, and I know how much they need food.

I go to the garage to feed Maya's pet rabbit, Dave. Maya follows me like a lost little dog. I hold her hand and ask her what we should choose for tea. It distracts her and we pick out a small M&S pizza for Jackson, which he will have with cucumber on the side. We'll make a chicken wrap for Maya and there is leek and potato soup for Macy, who became a vegetarian last year. I also get something small to eat as I feel light-headed.

Phil Daly, the brilliant press officer for the Leeds Rhinos calls in so that I can check the wording of the official club statement announcing Rob's death. It's word perfect and the announcement is made at 6pm.

Early evening passes peacefully. My phone is off, as is the television, and I have no idea that Rob's death is receiving blanket coverage on the main news and sports channels as an outpouring of love and grief elevate the internet.

I am oblivious to all of this and, once my mum and dad have left, I get the kids ready for bed. They are shattered. I tuck Jackson up in his little bed and his eyes close as I kiss him goodnight.

Macy and Maya are waiting for me outside his room. They look gorgeous in their summer pyjamas. They have a question for me. Can they sleep with me tonight?

I look at them and smile. 'Of course,' I say. 'Yeah, of course you can.'

An hour later with the girls curled around me, asleep in the dark, I give in to my own exhaustion. I think of Rob and before long I am also asleep, and at peace.

11

A Feather from Rob

Monday 3 June 2024, Pontefract

The car is strangely quiet at first. I know this is natural. Today is the first day of life without Rob. I am driving the children to school in a scenario that seemed unimaginable just twenty-four hours ago. At the hospital, as we faced the last few hours of Rob's life, the girls asked me a simple question: 'Do we have to go to school tomorrow?'

I took care to reassure them. 'No, of course not,' I said. 'It's okay to have time off. You definitely don't have to go to school.'

If we had not looked so sad, and he had not been dealing with so many new emotions all at once, I think Jackson might have done a tiny fist-pump and exclaimed: '*Yes!*'

We didn't mention school the rest of that long day. It was only in the evening, about an hour before we all went to bed, that Macy and Maya came to find me. Macy spoke first. 'Mum,' she said, 'I do want to go to school tomorrow.'

'Me too,' Maya said.

I looked at them carefully. 'Are you sure?'

They nodded in unison and we all hugged. I did feel for poor

Jackson as he had not been given much choice. His big sisters had made their decision and I backed them. In that moment it felt right. The girls were so clear about going to school, and trying to get back to normal, that it would have been hard for Jackson to stay at home on his own with me.

'All right,' I said. 'We'll go to school tomorrow.'

Jackson didn't protest, and I called my mum to tell her of the change in plan. Mum immediately said that she and Dad would take the children to school, but I was adamant. I would do it. I knew it would be hard going back for the first time. But it would still be difficult even if I waited until the following week. It was best I faced the sympathetic and curious faces of the other parents and children now.

Mum and Dad still wanted to help. Mum said that they would come round in the morning to work on our neglected garden. I was too tired to argue; I also accepted Mum's offer to call Mrs Carr, the assistant head teacher at Maya and Jackson's school.

I emailed Macy's head teacher and explained that she wanted to go to school, and that I supported her decision. The reply arrived quickly. It was full of compassion. The head stressed that the school would look after Macy and all her teachers would be informed. The family support liaison officer would also be at school, and they were all ready to talk to Macy whenever she wanted.

Both schools have shown such care throughout the past year – especially since Rob was hospitalised with his first bout of pneumonia. The children are in safe hands today.

But now, as the car moves closer and closer to the school gates, my heart aches for Macy. I know how much she feels the loss of her dad. This morning, when she came down for breakfast, Macy was worried about getting upset at school. I told her that it was totally normal if she wanted to cry. No one would think badly of her. If anything, people would almost expect her to be upset and there were plenty of adults who would talk kindly to her.

Macy's real concern was that she would become distressed in front of her friends. I reminded her that she has such lovely friends, and that if it becomes too much for her, the school will call me and I will be round in ten minutes to pick her up. She looked more cheerful while eating her breakfast and then packing her bag.

She is pale and silent now as we see the school ahead of us. I want to tell her that we can turn around and drive home. But I know that she needs to get through this first day. We all do.

Outside the school we feel a surge of relief. A small group of Macy's close friends are waiting for her. My big, brave girl smiles as I give her a quick hug and a kiss. Maya shouts her goodbye and then Macy is out of the car and inside the soothing huddle of her friends. I see a big bar of Dairy Milk chocolate and some squishy sweets being handed to her. Macy is smiling and I let slip a relieved sigh. I know she will be fine today.

As we drive on Maya chats away to me while Jackson has brought the worry worm the nurses gave him at the hospital. It calms him. They seem ready to go back.

But I feel vulnerable as we near the primary school. It is more difficult here. Rather than dropping off Maya and Jackson, as I do with Macy, I have to park the car and then queue outside the gates before walking them through the playground. That crowded space fills me with dread now. I can imagine everyone looking at us with pity in their eyes, moving aside to let us pass in silence and grief. Even worse, I picture a scene where mums I barely know walk up to me outside the school so they can talk and offer an awkward embrace. I know that everyone will mean well but today it will be too much. I will break down and cry helplessly if anyone says anything to me.

What good will I be then if Maya and Jackson see me in such a state?

I just want to take them to their classrooms and make sure their friends and teachers are there. And then, without a word to anyone else, I want to get home.

Of course there is no need for any of these jumbled anxieties. Everyone is really respectful. I am given space to concentrate on Maya and Jackson and no one interrupts us. I am able to talk calmly to the kids. They soon leave me for their friends and their classes.

I turn away and, suddenly feeling the weight of sadness, my head lowers. I walk quickly, looking down at the playground. It feels as if my mouth is about to crumple but I keep going, walking to the car. I am crying by the time I slide behind the wheel. I give myself a minute and then, blinking away the tears, I start the engine.

It sounds very matter-of-fact but I have already drawn up a

list of everything I need to do today. I am surprised there is so much paperwork and so many calls to make after a death. But, in a way, being practical and ticking off the jobs to be done will muffle my sorrow for a while.

Mum and Dad are already waiting for me by the time I get home. They have brought a shovel and some secateurs for their gardening. I wave aside their concern and tell them I am fine. I don't need to sit down and talk. I just want to get on with my tasks for the day. They worry about me, but they understand when I say this is the best way for me to cope.

Dad tells me he will cut the grass first while Mum does some clearing and tidying. I nod numbly and say that I will be on the phone. I've already spoken to the funeral directors and they will pick up Rob's body this morning. But they need the papers to be signed by the consultant, who is wonderfully kind to me when we talk on the phone. She wants to discuss the wording on the death certificate. Should we say that the cause of death was motor neurone disease?

I point out that pneumonia should be mentioned because Rob was being treated for that infection and it resulted in him being brought to hospital almost a week ago. But of course MND was the ultimate cause of his death. We decide that both aspiration pneumonia and MND should be written on the death certificate.

I don't like all this cold administration, but the hospital has given me a leaflet that lists all the government and financial organisations I need to contact to inform them of Rob's death. Other random tasks jump into my head and I am just about to cancel the blue badge that has allowed us to park in disabled bays when I see another message on my phone. There have been hundreds and I've not opened many of them. But I can see that this new one, at 8:54am, is from Prince William's communications officer. I read it in surprise:

> Lindsey, please don't reply to this, but just a message to say on behalf of all of us at Kensington Palace, that you and the family are in our thoughts. We were all so sorry to hear the news yesterday. Sending strength and love. Lee.

Mark, my brother, arrives. He has come to check on me and to make sure that Mum and Dad don't work too hard in the garden. It's good to see him, as always, and I take a break. After he is reassured that I am okay, Mark asks me if I watched the news last night and this morning. I haven't switched on the television since we've been back and so I am astonished when Mark tells me that Rob's death has been the main item on every single news broadcast for the last fifteen hours. He has seen moving and detailed coverage of Rob's life on *BBC Breakfast*, where our friends Claire Ryan and Sally Nugent have done so much in telling our story.

There are so many other tributes that I do the most sensible thing under the circumstances. I switch on the kettle and ask Mark to call my parents inside. I spoon coffee into four mugs and wait for the water to boil.

I miss Rob and think how I would love to get a message from him more than anyone: *Could I also have a coffee please, darling?* It would feel so peaceful to sit next to Rob, holding his cup while he drinks through a straw and I chat away about all the famous people who are talking about him.

The water rolls to a boil and I hear Mum, Dad and Mark. I soon join them in the front room and see that a red dot is shining on the television box. Rob used to record *BBC Breakfast* on a series link, which continues even though he is gone. He liked to watch the programme after he woke up, but of course today's show, like all the others from the past two weeks, will never be seen by him.

We watch some of the coverage while chatting over coffee. After Mum and Dad go back out into the garden, I am happy to sit a little longer with Mark. An hour goes past; I am only aware of the time when Mum pops back into the room.

'How come your coffee break's still going while we're sweating away outside?' she jokes. 'Me and your dad are sixty-five, you know.'

I know she is relieved that I have stopped and taken time out with Mark. But I still have a 101 things to do and I am soon back on the phone and my computer as I tick off one job after another. Life, even amid death, has to go on.

After school the following afternoon I drove the kids to Headingley so that we could look at the tributes that had been left for Rob. The home of the Leeds Rhinos was a sea of flowers and rugby shirts, handwritten messages and candles, blue-and-amber scarves and toy rhinos. It was beautiful but almost overwhelming to see such love, admiration and respect on display.

Phil Daly, the communications manager of the Rhinos, had warned me that there would be cameras at the ground. I said it was okay for us to be filmed and photographed looking at the tributes as it was important for people to see our appreciation for their messages. But I didn't want to be interviewed or speak on camera in case I broke down.

We then drove across to Seacroft Hospital in Leeds so that I could give some flowers to Dr Agam Jung who had looked after Rob so thoughtfully since early 2020. They got on brilliantly and it had meant the world to Rob and me that £6 million of the money we had raised would build a care centre in his name at Seacroft. The day after his death, the first spade had dug into the ground to start building the Rob Burrow Centre for Motor Neurone Disease.

Geoff, Irene, Joanne and Claire, as well as Kevin Sinfield, had all attended that ceremonial dig, hosted by Dr Jung. A day later it was our turn to be shown around the site by the lovely Dr Jung. It was tangible proof that Rob's legacy would live on, in the most practical and useful way, long after his death.

I still knew how important it was for the children to retain a sense of normality and so that evening they went to their swimming lessons. I had been worried about Macy as she had not eaten much the last two days and she was complaining of a tummy ache. But on the drive home from swimming, she, Maya and Jackson were cheerful. The car was full of chatter as we headed back to Pontefract.

As soon as I opened the front door, Maya came scampering in after me. 'Daddy,' she yelled happily, 'we're home!'

She suddenly stopped and, as she remembered that Rob's room was empty, the terrible truth hit her all over again. She burst into tears. I held her close, feeling determined that I would protect the children with all the love I had inside me.

The days passed and I felt Rob's absence acutely. I kept waiting for his machine to kick into gear and the next voice note to arrive. I yearned to hear Rob ask me for a Red Bull or to change the TV channel. I also longed for that feeling of being run off my feet as, beyond looking after the children, so much of my time had been devoted to caring for Rob.

I missed him and found the silence hard to bear. Even though we had not had a proper conversation for a long time I also missed the sound of my own voice talking to him. He was no longer there to hear me chatting away or voicing out loud any worries I had. There was just a hushed emptiness to the house when the kids were at school. I felt very alone.

Towards the end of that first week without Rob I spent an hour clearing stuff we had accumulated in the garage. As I walked back into the front room, I saw a little white feather right next to Rob's chair.

I stared at it. I knew it had not been there when I'd gone into the garage. *Rob*, I said softly in my head, *is that you?*

Of course anyone else would think I was just being silly because feathers float down all the time without us really noticing them. But this felt real. It felt like a sign from Rob. After all, a few weeks before I had asked Rob to try and send me a sign, if he could, to let us know that he was still with us. It was one of our poignant little jokes – just like Rob saying he hoped that he could become a ghost who would watch over us.

I took a photograph of the feather on my phone and then, carefully, I picked it up. My fingers curled around the feather to keep it safe.

Later, I googled the apparent meaning of a fallen white feather. I am not a particularly religious or spiritual person, but I found comfort in the online articles suggesting that it signified a link to a place existing outside our physical world. I lingered over a few lines in particular, which claimed that finding a fallen feather offered 'a connection to spiritual realms. Coming from birds, feathers symbolise freedom, both mental and physical, from the bounds of the earth.'

Logically, I know this is meaningless. But I want to believe it's true. I want to believe that my tiny feather is a message from Rob.

I feel Rob is still watching over us and, more than ever, I want to make him proud.

Slowly, I began to catch up with all the texts, emails and voice notes sent to me, as well as reading and watching some of the thousands of tributes to Rob. Grief can be debilitating and isolating but there were constant reminders of how Rob had touched the world. I could not feel stricken or alone with my pain when the love for and pride in Rob rolled on in wave after wave.

That Saturday afternoon, 8 June 2024, just six days after

our lives changed for ever, the Men's and Women's Challenge Cup Finals were both played at Wembley. Leeds were in the women's final, against St Helens, while Wigan and Warrington faced each other in the men's final. Wembley had been turned into a shrine for Rob.

His shirt number – 7 – was painted on the halfway line above the hashtag of #OneRobBurrow. Rob's gentle reminder, 'In a world full of adversity we must still dare to dream', was stitched into every player's jersey. During the warm-ups, all four teams wore the number 7 on their training shirts, while each of the female Rhinos carried the same number on their back in the final.

Outside the ground, fans from rival clubs laid flowers, shirts, scarves, blue balloons festooned with the number 7, and photographs of Rob adorned with handwritten messages to my husband. Each match was preceded by a long and immaculate silence, in honour of Rob, followed by sixty seconds of emotional applause.

The men's final began at exactly 3:07pm, while another minute of applause also reverberated around a packed Wembley in the seventh minute of the game – just as it did after seven minutes of the Premiership rugby union final that afternoon between Northampton and Bath at Twickenham. The children and I watched the Wembley game at home on television with a sense of wonder that their dad, my Rob, could have had such an impact on so many people.

I also liked the image of a giant banner draped across the entrance of Wembley Park Underground station. Above a photograph of Rob's smiling face there was a simple, resonant message: 'A lad from Yorkshire who got to live out his dream.'

Rob's favourite number 7 was again in my thinking as we planned his funeral. I wanted the service to take place on a Sunday, an unusual day for a funeral but one that is mostly free of rugby league fixtures – it was important that we included many former Rhinos. A Sunday was also our preference because I had been advised that, owing to Rob's profile, we needed security to ensure that only invited guests, rather than the media or strangers, could attend. It would be less intrusive for other families, too, not to have their ceremonies overlap with ours.

As it always takes time to arrange a funeral, it soon became apparent that an evocative date might be possible. The seventh of July, giving us a 7/7 anniversary, would have appealed to Rob so I was happy when the Pontefract crematorium confirmed its availability that day. They also were flexible in stressing that we could have as long as we liked as there would be no other services on the seventh. On a normal weekday, one funeral followed another and so a Sunday service felt like a true godsend.

Sunday 7 July 2024, Pontefract

The cortege slows to a crawl. I sit with Geoff, Irene, Macy, Maya and Jackson in the first car behind the hearse. My anxiety about the funeral, and how it will impact the children, is briefly dispelled by the sight of the massed crowds who have turned out to line the streets from our home to the crematorium. Eddie, the kind but slow-moving funeral director, tells me that around 20,000 people have gathered to show their respects and say goodbye to Rob.

I am struck by all the different rugby shirts. Fans from Castleford, Featherstone, Wakefield and Leeds stand together as an ancient and bitter rivalry is cast aside in memory of Rob. No one would normally wear a Leeds shirt in Castleford but today there can be no enmity because of the love everyone felt for him. People want to wear their colours to show how much Rob, and the way he played the game and lived his life, meant to them and their towns and teams.

The crowd is like an unending sea with wave after wave of people. Some place a flower on the black hearse, or simply touch the back of the car where the coffin is carried.

We are all amazed by the turnout but Macy, softly, asks this piercing question of Rob's illness and death: 'Why did it have to be my dad?'

I try my best to comfort her and her younger sister and brother and explain how proud we should be that their dad was so loved. But that unanswerable question worries me even more. How will Macy and Maya find the courage to stand up in the crematorium and deliver the first eulogies?

It takes us an hour to travel the two and a half miles from our house. When we turn in to the grounds of the crematorium, passing the small group of photographers who have been waiting so long, my heart begins to race. I can only wonder what my two lovely girls and boy feel in this moment of our family catastrophe.

We climb out of the car, feeling the compassionate gaze of sixty guests settle on us, and I try to gather Macy, Maya and Jackson around me. It helps that Lesley, the humanist celebrant, is waiting for us. She smiles and takes my hand. We wait for the pall-bearers to bring out the coffin. It is almost time.

But, first, little Jackson jumps when there is a high-pitched cry behind us. Kylie Leuluai, Rob's teammate for nine seasons, is a New Zealand prop of Samoan heritage. He messaged me a few days ago to ask if it would be appropriate for him and the other players of Māori or Polynesian Island heritage to perform a haka in tribute to Rob.

The haka throws down a mighty challenge to an opponent before battle while celebrating the spirit of an indigenous people. Rob had faced the haka before when he was named as the player of the tournament in Great Britain's series of internationals against New Zealand in 2007. He knew what it was like, even at a mere five foot five, to look up at the giants of New Zealand as they stomped their boots, slapped their thighs, beat their chests and waggled their tongues in a kind of war dance while hollering their proud words.

I knew how much Kylie meant to Rob. Kylie, after all, suffered more than anyone when Rob played his pranks on his fellow Rhinos. Kylie could have murdered Rob cheerfully on numerous occasions, but he loved him too much. So to have Kylie and his rugby-playing brothers do the haka as Rob's coffin approaches the crematorium carries a profound meaning of friendship and respect. I hold Jackson close as Kylie and the others begin to cry out:

> '*Ka mata, ka mata! Ka ora, ka ora!*
> *Ka mata, ka mata! Ka ora, ka ora!*'

In English this means:

> *It is death, it is death! It is life, it is life!*
> *It is death, it is death! It is life, it is life!*

Jackson stares in fascination as men born on the other side of the world show us how much Rob means to them as a fellow rugby warrior and close friend.

It helps to distract us but, soon enough, as the last cries of Kylie fade into a sombre silence, the moment arrives. It is time for the children and I to lead everyone into the crematorium. I smile at them and whisper encouraging words.

But the sight of the coffin, covered in flowers, makes us pause. It is too much for Maya and she cracks open. My little girl begins to sob. Her crying is so painful and so loud that I cannot see how she can join Macy at the front and read her words. But it doesn't matter if she can't get the words out. All that matters is that I try and comfort her.

I hold her tight and tell her that everything will be okay. I manage to help her take in some deep breaths and, gradually, her jagged crying softens and eases. She wipes her eyes and nods when I ask her if she feels better. She also nods when I ask if she still wants to try and join Macy at the front. And then, with the kind of courage that typifies their dad, Maya stands up and Macy leads the way. I am just floored by the character of my girls.

It is beyond me to talk at the funeral but, somehow, here they are, willing to raise their young voices in honour of the father they have just lost.

My pounding heart could break; I'm so worried. But there is no need. A strange composure envelopes both girls.

Maya looks up at us. Her voice rings out, clearly and beautifully:

'Thank you, everyone, for joining us to celebrate the life of our amazing dad. Today is a sad day, but it's a day to remember how special and loved our dad was.'

Macy steps forward to continue:

'To Maya, Jackson and I, he was simply the best dad in the world. He was our number one fan. He would often rush off after training to come and pick us up, take us to our after-school clubs and he would give us treats when Mum said no. He always had a smile on his face, especially when listening to Michael Jackson, drinking caffeine or watching the NFL.'

Gentle laughter ripples around the crematorium and I smile again at the girls. Macy keeps talking:

'Our dad has always been a true inspiration throughout his life, whether that was on the rugby field or during his battle with MND. He taught us how precious life is and to always live life to its fullest.

'Thank you for being our dad and for looking after us. You are without doubt the most bravest, loved dad in the whole world. I hope I grow up to be just like you.'

Her big sister's words give little Maya even more strength and, incredibly, her voice also fills the crematorium with love as she says:

'We love you, Dad, and we miss you, but we know that you will be with us every step of the way.

'Daddy, you will continue to inspire us every day and we will do our best to always make you proud.

'You'll always have a special place in my heart.'

I could burst with pride as applause breaks out and the girls walk back to the front pew to sit with me and Jackson. They look at me questioningly, but can soon tell how well they have done when I whisper my praise and smile helplessly at them.

Lesley moves to the front. 'Welcome to this special service,' she says. 'It's one amongst many times of paying tribute to Rob Burrow, except this is different. Today is not for the world. It's for his family and his good friends and the people closest to him. It's a time we will hear more personal tributes from his family and, of course, his friends. But this is a time for them to really express what Rob meant to them. There's no press, no cameras. It's just a sharing of memories and experiences with Rob, and they are words spoken from the heart.

'There probably isn't anything that hasn't already been said about Rob as a sportsman, as a humanitarian, as a fundraiser, as a hero. But we will hear some things that you haven't heard before. What better way could we have started than with Macy and Maya opening our service, with the first words coming from the family. And didn't they just do their dad proud, and their mum? Because let's not forget that before Rob was a rugby giant, metaphorically speaking, he was a son, he was a grandson, he was a brother and he was a much-loved husband and daddy. But before we hear family words, let's hear about some other aspects of Rob.'

Danny McGuire, Barrie McDermott, Jamie Jones-Buchanan and Kevin Sinfield take turns to speak. Each captures different strands of Rob's character. Danny remembers their friendship and unbreakable bond after playing alongside each other for twenty-five years, from juniors to battle-scarred veterans winning yet another grand final together. 'We will miss you, my mate,' Danny says in closing, 'and I know I say that on behalf of everyone who had the honour and pleasure of playing alongside you.'

Barrie describes the high jinks and riotous humour Rob brought to the dressing room. He has the crematorium rocking when refusing to detail Rob's most infamous party trick in the shower.

'If you know, you know,' Barrie says wryly.

After he has also paid more serious tribute to Rob, and kindly to me, Barrie has us all laughing again as he ends by saying: 'Like many others in this room it was my absolute honour to be your teammate and your friend, and it was my privilege to be your victim. I just hope you're up there doing what you do best, drinking copious amounts of Red Bull and showing David how to make Goliath cry. And when that Judas fellow takes a shower, you do your stuff, pal.'

Jamie is moving and philosophical as he outlines seven lessons and gifts of Rob's life. He ends by saying to Rob: 'With the life you lived, the example you set and the legacy that you left behind, I want you to know that despite being the smallest player of our generation, you always occupied the biggest part of our hearts. Thank you, you little giant.'

I hope Jamie doesn't mind but as soon as he finishes talking, Maya and I race to the toilet. She has been busting and holding on since lesson four of Jamie's eulogy – but we make it back in time for Kev's tribute.

Of the four friends, Kev finds it hardest to speak. He has run so many torturous marathons on behalf of Rob and MND so he understands physical pain and exhaustion better than any of us. Kev has also just flown all the way from New Zealand, where England's rugby union team are playing a Test series, and he will fly all the way back again tomorrow. It is yet another example of Kev's endurance and commitment – but I can see how tough this is for him.

Kev told me how he thinks so much about Rob every day. He could be out for a run and wherever he looks he sees the number 7 – whether on a car registration or the front of a house. Sometimes he would look at his watch and just say a breathless 'wow' because it told him that he had run 7.7 miles.

'Just over four and a half years ago Rob was diagnosed with MND,' Kev says. 'He accepted it. He wanted no fuss. He continued to smile every day in the face of adversity. I knew he was tough and I knew he was brave. And certainly he was special. However, throughout his MND journey, he became tougher, braver and more special than anyone I've ever known.

'Rob was part of our team as we've already learned today. But he became a special part of a different team after his MND diagnosis. This was Team MND. Rob changed the landscape for MND across the UK and influenced and inspired people all over the world. He had the courage to open his very private, beautiful and loving family life and never shied away from any event that would help the cause. He helped vulnerable people feel safe, feel accepted, brought them together and gave them a sense of belonging. People across the UK showed Rob's new team that they were valued, respected and loved. What a legacy.

'Some of you may not know this, but Rob used to play the Al Pacino *Any Given Sunday* speech to himself before games. He would walk around the dressing room in his pants and his headphones. He loved it.'

Kev reads a short extract of the speech and then explains why: 'Rob fought for a reason. He showed us what living and loving looks like and he always did this with the biggest smile. Over the last four happy years we became very close and I'll miss him dearly. I'll miss his dry sense of humour, the spark in his eyes, and, most of all, his big smile. Rob will continue to inspire in every single way and I will never forget the special times we shared, both on and off the field. Rob wanted those living with MND now, and those diagnosed in the future, to be able to be looked after properly. We want to find a cure.'

Lesley then delivers her own tribute to Rob and plays a video of the Pacino speech in full. She turns next to the family and, on a beautiful pre-recorded video, Geoff reads a poem he's adapted in honour of his beloved son. Joanne and Claire are funny and touching and then, near the end, Lesley reads the words I have written for Rob:

Dear Rob

If there is such a thing as soulmates, I would like to think that is us. We were two halves of a whole. Opposites that became a perfect match. You were the laid-back to my 'get stuff done'. The on time to me always being late. You were the heart of our family and I will hold up your half now – for you.

There are no words that could ever truly prepare me for when this time came because we always lived in hope that it never would. What I would give for one last hug, or to hear your machine: 'Can I have a Red Bull, darling?'

If only there were more Rob Burrows in the world, what a world that would be.

I promise you I will do you proud in everything I do.

Not all superheroes wear capes. Rob, you will forever be my hero, my one true love.

I love you more today than yesterday but nowhere near as much as tomorrow.

Love
Lindsey

The children keep looking at me, to make sure I am all right, and I manage to smile rather than cry. But I come close to breaking when a montage of photographs is shown on the big screen – of Rob looking young and gorgeous. We see him playing rugby and with me on holidays, before we married, and then at our wedding and with the children. The mosaic of memories is a reminder of how blissfully happy we were – which makes our loss feel so cruel now.

I bite my lip and blink hard before whispering to the children that it will soon be time to leave. But, first, we watch each member of the congregation say their own personal farewell to Rob as his favourite song, Michael Jackson's 'Man in the Mirror', resounds. The Rhinos lead the way, standing in a long line so that each of them can reach out and touch the coffin. Some of these giants of men bring their fingers to their lips, in a small kiss, before they then rest their hands briefly on the casket. They do so with such care and delicacy that I could cry helplessly. But I need to hold myself together for the sake of the children.

We are the last to leave and it feels unbearably hard to say one final goodbye to Rob. But we make it to the car only for Maya to start crying yet more heartfelt tears. 'I want to go back and see my dad,' she says over and over. 'I want to go back and see my dad.'

Incredibly, the wake at Farmer Copleys gives us a beautiful few hours. We all relax a little and talk and even laugh together. It helps me to see everyone while the children eat so much that they look as if they might pop. I even manage to have a bite to eat myself, while so many people tell me it was an unforgettable service and that we have done Rob proud. These are the words I really need to hear.

We get home around eight o'clock, feeling exhausted. While Maya and Jackson brush their teeth sleepily, Macy asks me a serious question: 'Why didn't you cry today, Mummy?'

I look at my big girl and feel a pang of regret. I have been so busy trying to look after the children that I've muffled my true feelings. I know she deserves an honest answer.

'I did cry a lot, on the inside, and at some points of the service,' I say. 'But I was so worried about upsetting you, Maya and Jackson. I tried to be brave for you because you were all so strong. I couldn't do what you and Maya did and stand up and read to everyone. I thought I would just start crying and not be able to stop. And that wouldn't have helped anyone.'

Macy listens intently and nods. 'But it's good to be able to cry at times like this,' I say. 'So you're right. I wish I had cried some more today.'

Stretching out her arms to me, Macy hugs me tight. 'You can always cry with us,' she says.

Rob was so positive and generous and, while he could still talk to me, he had once said: 'Lindsey, I don't want you to be sad when I'm gone. I want you to get on with your life. I want you and the kids to live the happiest and best possible life.'

Those words drive me now. I've got three beautiful children and Rob will live on in them. He might not be with us in person, but I will continue to try and make Macy, Maya and Jackson proud and happy. I will try to give them the best childhood. Even if he is no longer with us in person, I still feel Rob will be with me in a small way.

This belief is strengthened a few days after the funeral. The house is quiet and I come in from the garden on a sunny morning. I look across our front room and see another sign. A little feather has floated down on to the carpet right next to Rob's chair. It makes me smile.

'Hey, Rob,' I whisper. 'I miss you. But I'm doing okay, and the kids are great.'

I pick up the tiny feather, sit on the arm of his chair and feel grateful.

'Thank you,' I say softly.

12

Dare to Dream

In November 2023, seven months before his death, I had wheeled Rob down a long corridor lined with the ghosts of his past. The walls inside Headingley rugby ground were covered in giant photographs of special moments and great victories for the Leeds Rhinos. A younger version of Rob lit up many of the images.

As his chair rolled down the passageway, the wheels making a soft whirring sound on the blue floor, we passed a team photograph from fifteen years before. Rob, in his twenties, glowed with fitness and health, his pale blue eyes glinting in anticipation of all the glory that still lay ahead of him and the Rhinos.

I pointed out the next photograph too so that, hunched over and helpless in his chair, Rob could raise his eyes to see himself beaming in 2015, pointing his left arm skywards while his right hand rested on Kevin Sinfield's shoulder. Kev held the Super League trophy high on that unforgettable night at Old Trafford.

We headed for the dressing room and one photograph followed another. Rob was as static in his chair as those historic moments were frozen in their frames. But we loved seeing the joy and pride they captured as Kev rested the Challenge Cup on Rob's head. On we rolled, past Rob's clenched-fist salute after they had beaten Manly, the Australian champions in the 2012 World Club Challenge. We approached a blue-hued portrait of him and Danny McGuire, their smiling faces gleaming with sweat, rain or maybe a shower of champagne as they paraded the Super League trophy they had won in their last ever game for the Rhinos just six years earlier.

Near the end of the line there was a more sobering photograph from January 2020. It was taken just before the testimonial Jamie Jones-Buchanan shared with Rob a month after we had received his shattering diagnosis of MND. Jamie, looking straight into the camera, is typically dignified and serene. Standing behind him a pensive Rob, reeling and broken inside, looks down. Further back we see a thoughtful Danny McGuire, a sombre Kev, a reflective Kylie Leuluai and then, at the end, a regal and greying Jamie Peacock leaning against a white wall next to a battered, bald and somehow majestic Keith Senior.

All those great friends and teammates shared so much rapture and pain on the pitch, and they supported Rob through his harrowing years of MND. In the photograph they were about to walk out for the last time together for an elegiac tribute game against the Bradford Bulls. Eight months later Rob would no longer be able to walk.

I wondered what thoughts spooled through my husband's

mind as I turned the wheelchair into the deserted dressing room in which he and his friends had prepared for hundreds of games over the years. We were being filmed there by a BBC crew, as Rob prepared to say goodbye to the world, and the lighting was muted and suitably atmospheric. This sacred place for the Rhinos looked beautiful. The dark wood panels and benches seemed stately.

A solitary Rhinos jersey hung on a hook in the corner. It carried a number and name: 7 and Burrow made a perfect fit.

The silence was broken by the gentle clatter of Rob's wheelchair as it crossed the hard and shiny surface. So many drops of sweat, and occasionally blood, had fallen on that floor. Many times Rob had felt anxious and nervous there, asking Barrie or Kev if they thought he was good enough.

In the vast and empty room Rob's head tilted to the side as I wheeled him towards the centre. He used to walk intently around this space before a match, his headphones on as he listened to Al Pacino in *Any Given Sunday*. Rob would probably be in his underpants as Pacino's voice echoed in his head, telling him 'it all comes down to today . . . In any fight it's the guy who's willing to die who's going to win that inch.'

I felt even closer to Rob then as I brushed away the last crease in his new dark blue shirt and then, carefully, wiped his mouth with a cloth. The camera would be trained on him as the film began and his voice, resonating through the Eyegaze machine, would address the world in public for the last time.

I wanted Rob to look just right, a proud and gorgeous man right to the very end.

We had agreed to the request from the BBC to make one final documentary because they had stressed it would only be screened a few days after Rob's death. It would be a celebration of his life and, also, a tribute to everyone who fought against MND.

Just before Christmas in 2023, Rob and I were granted a private preview of the finished documentary. It was a profound and moving experience as we watched ourselves, not only from the month before but all the way through the years as Rob's life and subsequent struggles with the disease were spliced together.

The film began in the Rhinos dressing room with Rob alone in his chair, his eyes fixed on the Eyegaze screen in front of him as his computerised voice said: 'I hope one day we find a cure and live in a world free of MND. By the time that you watch this, I will no longer be here.'

As Rob and I sat together there was something so strange, yet tender, about knowing that other people would only see these scenes once he was gone. We felt proud too. The subject was hard, just like MND and life itself, and death was coming. But Rob never seemed lost or defeated – even when he explained the basic devastation of his condition: 'I'm a prisoner in my own body. That is the way MND gets you. The lights are on but no one is home. I think like you, but my mind doesn't work right. I can't move my body.'

Dr Agam Jung, our favourite neurologist, explained MND

with similar clarity: 'You may not be able to speak. You may not be able to swallow. You may not be able to breathe independently. And, of course, you can have weakness in your arms and legs and all of this leads to dependency and a reduced lifespan. It is a life-limiting condition.'

She also described the transformative impact that the Rob Burrow Centre for Motor Neurone Disease would have on so many patients at Seacroft Hospital in Leeds. But, then, Dr Jung said something extraordinary about Rob: 'I want to build this Rob Burrow Centre and he's supporting this. But that's not quite the legacy. Rob's legacy is how to live life in the now, against all odds.'

I saw the truth of those words all over again as, on screen, love and gratitude poured out of Rob as he said: 'I have had such a great life. I have been gifted with a wonderful wife and the most incredible three children. I hope that they know how much I love them.'

He added: 'I could not be any more proud of my kids. They are living their best lives and I couldn't ask for any more from them. I love my wife and kids more than anything. It kills me seeing Lindsey juggling everything because I was such a hands-on dad. You hate to see your wife with the burden of doing it alone. I think I would have broken down if it was me, but Lindsey has this unwavering patience with everyone.'

How could I be anything but patient while caring for the husband I loved, the gentle and funny and wise man who, in the very last minute of the film, said: 'I am just a lad from Yorkshire who got to live out his dream of playing rugby league.

As a father of three young children, I would never want any family to have to go through what my family and children have since my diagnosis. I hope I have left a mark on the disease. I hope it shows to live in the moment. I hope you find inspiration from the whole story. My final message to you is, whatever your personal battle, be brave and face it. Every single day is precious. Don't waste a moment. In a world full of adversity we must still dare to dream.'

In the documentary, as Rob shared his last resonant message with the world, my face filled the screen. You could see the pride and sorrow, grief and love, etched into my tangled features.

The camera then cut away to Rob's face. He looked suddenly amused as he paused.

I remembered how, with a horrified laugh, I had scolded him after I heard what he said next. I had exclaimed: 'Rob! You can't end it like that!'

But of course Rob knew best and he ended his final message to the world in his own lovely and witty way by saying: 'Rob Burrow, over and out.'

A delicious grin spread across his cheeky face before, finally, the screen turned black and the credits rolled.

Rob had been encouraging me to take the children to our villa in Florida for years. When he was too ill to even consider a brief holiday close to home, he urged me to have a break in America with Macy, Maya and Jackson. He knew they would love it but I was never going to leave Rob. It also wouldn't be fair to expect his parents to do everything while I was away.

I still worried about the children missing out and so, early in 2024, I allowed my parents to take them to Gran Canaria for a week while I stayed at home with Rob. America remained a distant dream.

There had been a time, with Covid seeming an endless nightmare, when I had tried to persuade Rob that we should sell the Florida villa. The insurance on the villa had run out and the renewal was extortionate. I told Rob that I would shop around and find us a more reasonable quote. But I was so busy looking after him and the kids that it slipped my mind. Soon afterwards there was a hurricane and the villa's roof got badly damaged. We were lumbered with a huge bill to fit a completely new roof.

It had been all my fault but I felt disillusioned as the villa was costing us so much money. We couldn't rent it out because of Covid and we were still paying management and maintenance fees. 'It's just not worth it,' I said. 'I think we should sell it.'

Rob was adamant. 'I want to keep the villa,' he insisted. I knew why. Rob had wanted us to spend part of our retirement out in Florida. That would no longer happen but another dream persisted. Rob wanted to leave the villa to the children and, eventually, to their own children in turn. It belonged to the whole family, not just us.

He was right and I could soon breathe a sigh of relief. Covid eased and bookings returned to their usual frequency and it made Rob happy to think that, one day, I would return with the children.

We had a late cancellation for early August 2024 and, rather than put the villa back on the rental market, I knew what Rob would want. Two months after his death we might begin to recover in the Florida sunshine, so I spoke to my parents and the children about our going out together. Everyone was excited and I became caught up in the anticipation.

I was exhausted; I hadn't had a break since the late summer of 2019. Part of me just wanted to close my eyes and stretch out in the sun but I also wanted to make it special for the kids. So I suggested that we spend a week at the villa and then go on a Disney cruise. The squeals of delight made me certain that I had done the right thing.

Once the booking was complete a small thrill rippled through me. We were going away. We were going to have an actual holiday again.

Those feelings did not last. I thought of Rob and felt guilty. I began to cry bitterly. How could I think of myself and be in the sunshine when Rob was dead? How could I feel any excitement when we had lost Rob for ever? How could I smile when thinking of something as indulgent as a holiday? How could I be so cold and insensitive?

It took a while but I calmed down and worked out what Rob would have said. He would have told me to stop being daft and think of how much the children and I needed time away.

We would fly from Gatwick to Florida and, as it was an early flight, I booked my parents, the kids and me into an airport hotel. Jackson loves trains so even the train journey from Pontefract down south was an exhilarating adventure for him. The girls also loved staying overnight at Gatwick and the six of us found it easy to get up before dawn the following morning.

We were just about to leave the hotel, which was a short walk from the terminal, when my phoned pinged with a deflating message: *Your flight has been cancelled.*

I couldn't believe it. I tried to be optimistic and thought we would probably fly a few hours later that morning. We trudged to the check-in desk where a long line of people were discovering the same news. There was a technical fault with our plane and we would actually not be flying for at least twenty-four hours while the airline tried to find everyone alternative flights.

The disappointment on the children's faces was painful to see. I did my best to sort something out and we were luckier than most of the passengers as six spare seats were found for us on the equivalent flight the next morning. We just had a day to kill.

At least, in compensation, we were being put up in a much swankier hotel than the night before, and all our meals were paid for. I still expected that I was in for a day from hell with three dejected kids. But they surprised me in the best possible way. We ended up having a fantastic time. It helped that the iPad kept them busy most of the morning as they played games and watched a movie. Then, in the afternoon, my parents stepped in to offer some old-fashioned entertainment. They took us for a walk around the perimeter of Gatwick Airport. Jackson was smitten by the sight of so many aeroplanes taking off and climbing high in the sky, while the girls loved blackberry-picking. We filled a small bag with blackberries, which were so delicious we devoured them all when we got back to the hotel.

The flight the following day went smoothly but we faced another test soon after we arrived at the villa. My phone pinged with another ominous message. We were warned that Hurricane Debby would hit land the next morning and that we would have to take shelter and stay indoors. Soon the winds were high and loud, and it rained heavily, but thankfully only the swimming pool netting was lost as Debby mostly skirted our villa. The hurricane had weakened into a slow-moving tropical cyclone and we avoided the worst of the damage. The kids were great, again, and there were no complaints as we hunkered down in the villa.

During the bad weather, Jackson played with his little camera, which allowed him to print out photographs. He didn't have much storage left and I told him he needed to delete some pictures. While he was quietly doing that he found some old photographs of Rob. He printed off five images and gave one each to me, his sisters and his grandparents.

'You've all got a picture of Daddy now,' he said proudly.

Everything settled down, the sun came out again and we had some joyful days at the Disney and Universal theme parks. I imagined how much Rob would have loved it as the girls, the two biggest adrenaline junkies I know, insisted on going on all of the biggest rides. Macy didn't miss out on any while Maya was mortified when she was told that she was too small for two of them. But she was allowed on the others because she just reached the one-metre-thirty height requirement.

The two of them loved the most terrifying rides and Maya insisted that she never screamed. I was happiest just waiting for them at the bottom – my level of adventure-taking saw me enjoy the Country Bear Jamboree with Jackson while the Seven Dwarfs Mine Train was as crazy as I got.

Rob, who had been Yorkshire's greatest Disney obsessive, would have been thrilled by our cruise, which we took a few days after the trip to the theme park. It was Disney all the way.

I had wondered if I would sometimes feel heartbroken being back at the villa and in Florida without Rob. There were some bittersweet moments, as I thought how much I missed him and how he would have loved being with us all. But it turned out to be a wonderful holiday filled with laughter and happiness.

Even before it was over we had decided we would return a year later with my brother, Mark, and his family. We all had the Rob Burrow bug for Disney, Florida and America.

We had only been back in Pontefract for five days when Macy, Maya and I found ourselves packing our bags for London. Jackson had zero interest in Taylor Swift and so he would happily spend the forthcoming weekend in Castleford with my parents. But the girls, two passionate little Swifties, were almost beside themselves with excitement as I had been given three tickets for one of her Wembley gigs.

It was a gorgeous summer evening and, after we had checked in at our hotel, we arrived early for the concert. By the time Taylor Swift arrived on stage my girls were in a beautiful frenzy.

For the next three and a half hours they didn't stop dancing while Maya didn't stop singing. She and Macy seemed to know every word of every song. Maya was just scandalised when I slipped to the loo and missed a couple of songs from *Reputation*, her favourite album. She and Macy were probably even more horrified when I started singing and dancing with them to 'Love Story'. They have always made it clear that I am the worst singer and most embarrassing dancer in the family. But they soon relented and allowed me to dance and sing along with them on an unforgettable night.

I realised all over again how lucky I am when Macy, Maya and Jackson were asked if they wanted to contribute to this book. I wasn't sure if this was a good idea at first as I didn't want them to feel that they were being forced to do something on my behalf. But the girls were immediately keen to be involved. They had to persuade Jackson, just a little, and he decided to use his five-year-old's artistic skills to paint me a lovely picture.

Macy, aged twelve, chose to write about me in the most thoughtful and generous way:

Resilient, kind and caring are the words that come to mind when I think about my mum. Her strength and courage inspire me to be strong. Through her selflessness and unwavering support, she has taught me the true meaning of love and family.

I admire my mum for how she looked after and cared for my dad throughout his illness. Always putting the needs of others before herself. It wasn't always an easy job. She constantly had to juggle looking after me and my siblings, being a full-time carer to my dad, as well as working part-time as a physiotherapist within the NHS. Her determination and devotion to helping others is what makes me most proud.

Mum was a beacon of strength, a source of comfort and a pillar of support during the most difficult times of our lives. As my dad once said, 'She is stronger than any rugby player I've ever played against.'

If I grow up to be a fraction of what you are, Mum, I know I will succeed in life.

Mum, you are so special and I hope you know how much Maya, Jackson and I appreciate everything that you have done for our family. We love you more than words can express.

Our mum's story is a reminder of the power of love, resilience and community support. Her unwavering dedication to her family in the face of adversity has been truly inspiring. Mum's strength, compassion and selflessness serve as a shining example of the incredible impact one person can have on those around them.

Macy

Nine-year-old Maya, meanwhile, wrote me a beautiful letter:

Dear Mum

I wanted to tell you how much I admire and look up to you. You are the best mum in the whole wide world, and I am so lucky to have you as my mum.

Every day, you put a smile on my face. You make me feel special and loved. I love spending time with you, whether we are playing games, reading stories or watching a movie together. I couldn't wish for a better mum.

You are always there for me, no matter what. Your hugs and kisses make everything better. You cheer me up when I am feeling sad. You've taught me about the importance of kindness, respect and honesty.

I love you more than you would ever know.

All my love
Maya

Macy, Maya and Jackson have helped heal my raw grief and given me renewed purpose. I am more determined than ever to give them the best possible life I can. Without them I am not sure how I would have coped. In the same way, I don't know how well I could have cared for Rob had I not received unstinting support from my parents, Rob's mum and dad and our friends. My brother and Rob's sisters, as well as so many members of the extended family, also helped when it sometimes felt as if I might buckle under the strain.

Six people a day are diagnosed with MND in the UK. The demands on those who care for anyone with the illness are harsh and relentless. The same difficulties apply to the millions of unpaid carers who look after their loved ones during other terminal or debilitating illnesses. My desire to highlight the often ignored stories of our carers has only intensified.

In the autumn of 2024, I reached my twentieth anniversary as an NHS physiotherapist. Caring for others, and trying to alleviate their pain, is built into my identity. I am intensely proud to work for the NHS but I have become increasingly dismayed and even angry with the way in which unpaid carers are treated in this country.

The statistics tell a stark story. Almost 10.6 million unpaid carers look after their ill or disabled relatives across the UK. As the population ages the demand for more carers is rising constantly. An estimated 600 people a day leave work to care for others. The pressures are vast: around two million unpaid carers in the UK are over sixty-five while the Joseph Rowntree Foundation has reported that 44 per cent of working-age carers are in poverty. Those figures are echoed by the MND Association, which has suggested that 47 per cent of unpaid carers looking after relatives with the disease are worried about money.

This contrast with my own privileged position has spurred me on to try and help shed light on the plight of so many of my fellow carers. In February 2024, I presented an ITV documentary called *Who Cares for Our Carers?* In the course of the programme I met numerous carers who were facing much more adversity than I had done. I was touched by the difficulties endured by Sue Ray, a 71-year-old woman whose husband, Norman, has dementia. Sue is a full-time carer for both Norman and her 98-year-old mum who also lives with them. Known as a 'sandwich carer', someone who looks after two people from different generations, Sue's fifteen-hour days begin at six every morning and are filled with cooking, cleaning, caring, doling out medication, running her house and paying the bills.

'I just want to have some peace,' Sue told me on camera. 'Not to be thinking about other people all the time.'

The same relentless demands also affected Chrissie, another woman I interviewed for the programme. She cares for her seventeen-year-old son, Alex, who was born with a rare genetic disorder, which means he can't talk or walk and has the developmental age of a baby. 'Your life stops,' Chrissie told me. 'I went from working full-time, having a social life, and that's it. It's gone. It's very isolating.'

Chrissie receives a carer's allowance of £76.75 a week, which was the lowest benefit of its kind. She told me: 'I'm on antidepressants. I've been on them for a number of years. You can go downhill quick.'

Fifty-nine per cent of carers in the UK are women – like Chrissie, Sue and myself – and there is a significant gender disparity. You have a 1 in 2 chance of becoming a carer by the time you turn fifty. But that age lowers to forty-six if you're a woman while it rises to fifty-seven if you're a man. That eleven-year disparity is just one of the many inequalities surrounding the unpaid care system.

When I heard the story of a man called Michael in Bradford, my understanding of the wider struggle for carers deepened. Michael cares full-time for his 29-year-old daughter, Susie, who has cerebral palsy and other conditions that mean she requires full-time care. 'Sometimes the day can start at four in the morning, if she's having a particularly bad night,' Michael said as he also outlined his battle with money.

He had given up work seventeen years before to care for Susie. His carer's allowance and other benefits were not enough to help him stay afloat during the cost-of-living crisis. 'Nearly every month I have more going out than I actually have coming in,' Michael said. 'Before the big price rises on gas and electric, I was already living in fuel poverty. I am using savings in order to pay my bills and buy the food.'

Michael explained that he needed something more than just economic support. 'What would make it better? Sometimes it can just be having somebody to talk to or somebody to come in to look after your loved ones so you can get out for a walk, or even take yourself off to your room and have a lie-down. That would all be a help.'

Michael's quiet anger was evident. 'It's such a dirty word,' he said of being a carer. 'This is what I've realised. I'm really proud of being a carer. I really am. I think it's one of the most honourable things you can offer another human being. The government definitely does not do enough. In terms of a job it's not valued at all.'

Helen Walker, the chief executive of Carers UK, told me: 'If every unpaid carer stopped caring tomorrow, our health and social care system would simply collapse. The value of their care is £162 billion. It's the same as a second NHS. We simply can't afford for people to stop caring.'

Yet so many carers are on their knees. Recent research found that only one out of every forty-two carers receives any 'respite care', a short-term break, from a few hours to a few weeks, that can enable them to rest and recharge. Some 470,000 carers seeking respite are waiting for an assessment from their local authority.

I never had to apply for any benefits or for respite care when I looked after Rob. But I have seen everything it entails, and I know I would have struggled with all the paperwork and the hurdles that need to be cleared just to get your case heard. I appreciate that every application needs to be vetted but the system seems skewed against the interests of the carers – even though they are essentially keeping much of the country going.

I'm not a confrontational person but I have become a passionate advocate for carers. That determination in me will only grow because, more than ever, I realise how much we need to take care of each other. I want the voices of carers to be heard and for the government to acknowledge the vital roles that they play in society.

I am proud to have been a full-time carer and I was fortunate to receive incredible kindness from so many people. Every carer in the country deserves the same respect and support that made my burden and pain so much easier to bear. That might seem an impossible dream. But, at such a dark and difficult time for the world, we should all hear Rob and dare to dream and try to make it happen.

For my children, of course, a holiday in America and a Taylor Swift concert cannot replace their dad. Macy, Maya and Jackson still struggle at times. There have been days when Maya has been upset. The boy at her school didn't mean to make her cry when he asked Maya if she still missed her dad: it was a perfectly innocent question but it hit a nerve.

We have found a way to help Maya and she now has a password at school. If she feels sad or stressed she will say the password and be taken to see Mrs Carr, the assistant head, who knows us so well. Mrs Carr and Maya sit down together and my little girl is soon back on an even keel.

Macy is sometimes quiet and thoughtful while Jackson still takes his worry worm with him wherever he goes. My dad recently picked him up from school and Jackson showed him the drawing he had done. When my dad complimented him, Jackson said: 'I think we should go to the hospital and show Daddy.'

My dad just smiled at him and said: 'That's a lovely thought, Jackson.'

So we are all learning to adjust to the loss and on 26 September 2024 we got through Rob's first birthday since his death. He would have turned forty-two.

I still catch myself thinking, *Oh, I must tell Rob.* Around the time of his birthday someone we knew passed away at the squash club and my first instinct was to message Rob and tell him: *Oh Rob, I can't believe it but Cliff's passed away.* Sometimes, as I leave the hospital in Leeds where I work part-time, I reach for my phone. I am just about to send Rob a text:

I'm on my way, darling. Love you xx.

Then, of course, the truth hits me again. Rob is gone and I pause in surprise that this is now the reality of my life.

But Rob is also loved and celebrated by the wider world and that remains a great comfort. A month before his birthday we were invited by Rhodri Jones of Rugby League Commercial to the Super League Grand Final to be played at Old Trafford in October. The Harry Sunderland Trophy, awarded to the Man of the Match, is now called the Rob Burrow Award. The children and I were asked if we would be willing to walk out with the new trophy, whose design we'd choose, before the match began. Rhodri then hoped that Geoff would present the trophy, in his son's name, to the winner.

Geoff was reluctant at first, as he felt it might be too overwhelming, but we all convinced him to accept. He knew that Rob would have loved him to present the award. Jackson was also a little shy about walking out in front of 70,000 spectators but he agreed that we would see how he felt on the day.

We were on our way to Manchester where their dad had won eight Grand Finals and two Man of the Match awards. It would be another night to remember.

Saturday 12 October 2024, Pontefract and Manchester

It's the usual rush to get everyone ready and out the door. Today is busier than usual as Jackson has been at football all morning, Macy at gymnastics and Maya with her friends, while I've just got back from having my hair cut. We've had a quick lunch, got dressed and now, at one-thirty, we're finally in the car. It's noisy and chaotic as I type Old Trafford into the satnav. The quickest route is chosen and I ease the car into gear.

We roll down our road and, with a sigh of relief, I switch on the radio.

The song is already halfway through but I almost slow to a stop in surprise. The achingly familiar sound of an old Black Eyed Peas track fills the car. It's been years since I last heard 'I Gotta Feeling' and so it is almost eerie that it should be playing on the radio just as we start our journey.

I am suddenly back in Manchester in 2011, before any of the kids were born, and these same cheesy words filling the car now boom around Old Trafford:

> *I gotta feeling*
> *That tonight's gonna be a good night . . .*

'Oh, just listen to this,' I tell the kids as I turn up the volume and they hear the echoing chorus that tonight's gonna be a good, good night.

They don't seem particularly interested until I start telling them how this song was played straight after the 2011 Grand Final, when their dad was the Man of the Match after scoring the famous try they have seen so often on YouTube. Rob told me that the Rhinos also played and danced to this same song on the bus from the stadium back to the hotel.

It seems incredible that, after not hearing it for so long, it should jump out of the radio at this very moment. Thirteen years have slipped by and our family has been formed by three births and scarred deeply by one tragic death. But I feel that, somehow, Rob is in the car with us now. He is no longer the sensational try-scoring master from that great night of the 2011 Grand Final but he is my Rob, and the kids' dad, and he calms and settles me as we get ready to cross the Pennines and honour him once more.

The miles pass and the journey is smooth until we hit traffic on the M62. The kids are hungry, yet again, and so I take the slip road so we can have a little break. We need petrol and I also become the most popular mum in the world again as I agree to buy them some Krispy Kreme doughnuts. The little break helps because the traffic has improved by the time we are back on the road. It's also bliss as the car is quiet while they tuck into their treat.

Two hours after we set off, we turn in to Old Trafford, just behind the luxury coach carrying the Hull KR players who will play Wigan Warriors this evening.

We are treated like royalty by so many kind people as we're whisked up into a box high in the stands. Everyone makes a fuss of the children, which is not quite what Jackson wants, and we're then given a lovely meal. Time flashes past and we are soon taken down into the bowels of the stadium and shown into a room where the Rob Burrow Award trophy is gleaming and waiting for us. It looks stunning and Macy points to the two engravings of her dad's name lower down as, in a lovely touch, they have listed the past winners of the Harry Sunderland Trophy around the bottom of the new cup.

Jackson is even less sure that he wants to walk out with his sisters in another ten minutes but we are distracted from our discussions and negotiations with him. We are shown the white gloves that the kids will wear when they carry the trophy on to the pitch. The gloves mean that they won't leave any Krispy Kreme-stained fingerprints on the cup – but they also give Maya a chance to do her impersonation of Michael Jackson. She brings her white-gloved hand to her bowed head and breaks out into a backward-strutting moonwalk. I can't help but laugh as I wonder what Rob would have said if he could have seen his little girl dancing like Michael Jackson, just minutes before she walked out at a sold-out Old Trafford.

I'm not sure we are going to win the battle to persuade Jackson to join the girls out on the pitch as he seems deeply uncertain. 'Let's see how you feel in a minute,' I suggest diplomatically.

He looks very smart in his little navy blue jacket. The girls, meanwhile, are beautiful as they hold up the trophy in a practice session while I take some photos on my phone. Macy wears an elegant blue dress with yellow and white trim, while Maya looks very swish in her new coat.

They can't stop smiling and their confidence and excitement sweep away the remaining doubts in Jackson. When I ask him again if he would like to go out with the girls he smiles and nods. Macy and Maya cheer and they are ushered to the front of the tunnel. I follow close behind, my heart swelling.

Maya's white-gloved right hand holds one side of the Rob Burrow Award while Macy, also wearing one white glove on her left hand, holds the other side. Jackson is to the right of his big sister and he has broken out into some kind of surreal routine. It's definitely not the moonwalk – more of a skittish jitterbug interspersed with jumps and skips. All that matters to me is that he looks happy.

They are just about to be given the signal to walk out when I notice evidence of the chocolate pudding Jackson has just eaten upstairs. I lean across to wipe the chocolate away from the corner of his mouth and remind him to smile.

I do it just in time: the music starts and Macy takes Jackson by the hand as she and Maya, holding the trophy named after their dad, walk out as sustained and emotional applause rolls across Manchester United's Theatre of Dreams. I keep taking photos as they move across the pitch to one of our favourite songs – 'One Call Away' by Charlie Puth. I am amazed that the photos are actually in focus because my eyes are so full of tears.

Fireworks shoot into the early evening sky. People are standing now, roaring as well as clapping as they watch our three smiling children. Above them the big screen is lit up by a photograph of their dad.

'Special, special people, with a special father,' the commentator on Sky Sports says to Sam Tomkins, the great former rugby league player who faced Rob so many times when Wigan went into battle against the Rhinos.

'Absolutely,' Sam says. 'I think the reception these children are getting now is testament to what a great man Rob was and how much he has done for the sport. Rob gave so many people so many great memories on this pitch.'

The children reach the blue plinth. Macy takes the other side of the trophy from Maya and, carefully, she places it in the right spot. She then leans down to check that Jackson and Maya are both doing okay. He just beams at her and jumps up and down while Maya bites her lower lip in an effort to control the width of her own smile.

'Those girls, and little Jackson, every time I see them I am blown away, Jon, by what they've achieved.' the commentator says to Jon Wilkin, the former St Helens star who also played against Rob so many times.

'Yeah, it's immense bravery from his whole family in the face of adversity,' Jon says, 'particularly his wife and his parents as well. They've just showed a real stoic grit – maybe something that the modern world doesn't see often enough.'

Macy, hand-in-hand with her sister and brother, turns to walk back the way they have just come.

'Oh, the roar that has come up for them . . .' the commentator says.

I hug them tight, showering kisses on my two girls and boy, but we need to move quickly to reach our seats in the stands.

We sit just in front of Geoff and Mike, my brother-in-law who is married to Rob's sister Claire. Geoff and Mike give the children a huge welcome and tell them how well they have done.

So much emotion swirls through me and, with everyone settled and safe, I take a deep breath as the whistle blows to start the match. I look up, for just a moment, and I nearly cry out as I see it floating towards me.

A little feather twirls slowly down as I gaze at it in wonder. The floodlights make it glow in the dark and I can't believe what I am seeing.

'Mike,' I exclaim. 'Look, the feather . . .'

I point as it drifts closer and closer. Mike looks and then laughs. 'That's Rob . . .'

It's become a standing joke on our family WhatsApp. Whenever anyone sees a feather, they report it on the group chat.

But I could almost cry now. I know it's just a feather but it really does feel like Rob is back with us. I catch the feather and hold it gently in my hand as the match unfolds in front of us.

It's a tough, low-scoring, attritional game but there is one moment of pure magic that even I, with my limited knowledge of rugby, can savour. Bevan French, the Australian who inspires this dominant Wigan team, steps off his right foot to dance through a gap before he repeats the same trick to blast open the Hull defence. His stunning try might not match the wonder score from Rob in 2011 – but it has Old Trafford rocking.

The rest of the match passes in a blur and, while no one else can tell, I am watching another game altogether in my head. It's a game full of those ghosts of the past as Rob shines in my imagination. All my memories of the Grand Finals I watched him play here reel through my mind. It's almost as if I am back there, with him, and we are just the young and giddy Rob and Lindsey, rather than the couple who endured MND together with the kind of stoicism that Jon Wilkin now sees in our children.

But there is such joy and love in Macy, Maya and Jackson, which means that they are far more than just brave little stoics. The final whistle blows and Wigan's 9–2 victory seals their incredible clean sweep of all four trophies this season – a feat that eluded the Rhinos at the height of their glory years. It is time for Geoff to be led down the stairs and out on to the pitch so that he can present the Man of the Match trophy.

'Go, Grandad, go!' the kids chant as Geoff, choked with emotion, leaves us.

I am also fighting back the tears when we eventually see Grandad Geoff hand over the inaugural Rob Burrow Award to Bevan French, the great young Australian who, in an eerie coincidence, lost his mum to MND two years ago.

Four months ago, in June, a week after Rob's death, Bevan also won the Lance Todd Trophy for his Man of the Match display at the Challenge Cup final at Wembley. That match was dominated by such heartfelt tributes to Rob and, afterwards, Bevan recalled how 'a couple of years ago I lost my mum to the same thing.' He went on, 'with Rob obviously being such a legend, it has connected to me a bit emotionally. It has made this week sweet, especially the fact that . . . the first trophy I won since I came back to England after she passed away was the Challenge Cup.'

Now, having become the first player to win Man of the Match awards at both the Challenge Cup and the Grand Final in the same season, Bevan is even more overcome to receive his trophy from Rob's dad. His emotions are heightened, too, as Wigan have flown his family from Australia and they surprised him on the eve of the final. Memories of his mum, and ours of Rob, are intertwined. There could be no better first recipient of Rob's new award.

It's after nine-thirty when we make it back to the car. I type our home postcode into the satnav and am just about to turn on the ignition when a sharp rap on my window makes me jump.

Keith Senior and Gareth Ellis, Rob's former teammates at the Rhinos, just want to say hello. It's great to see them and they tell the children how they have done their dad proud.

The Black Eyed Peas were right. It has been a good, good night and the kids are still flying as we cruise down the M62. Maya also has a new plan, which entails stopping at a McDonalds on the journey home. I feel happy and so I cause more cheers to erupt when I agree to one last treat for the night.

An hour later, after the chicken nuggets have been demolished, the car is quiet. The children are sleepy and I feel completely in the moment, right in the here and now, as all the pain of the last five years recedes a little further. The ghosts of the past are just beautiful memories of Rob which will keep him close to us for ever.

I can still feel his presence as we take the Pontefract turn-off. I feel all Rob's positivity and love and remember how he was devoid of self-pity. He showed us how to live and I see his example every day, and especially tonight, in Macy, Maya and Jackson. They are thriving and living their lives to the full, just as Rob always wanted them to do. I cannot wait to see what each of them goes on to achieve because I know they will make the most of every opportunity that comes their way.

I think of their dad, of Rob, the love of my life, as we drive the last few miles home. And I remember once again what he told us just before he said 'Rob Burrow, over and out' and the screen went black. Rob gave me, and all of us, these last words of courage and hope:

My final message to you is, whatever your personal battle, be brave and face it. Every single day is precious. Don't waste a moment. In a world full of adversity we must still dare to dream.

Acknowledgements

I would like to thank Ruth Cairns, my literary agent at Featherstone Cairns, for believing that I had a story to tell. Having been the literary agent for Rob's autobiography, *Too Many Reasons to Live*, Ruth has become a dear friend. Her help and guidance have been invaluable.

I really appreciate all the hard work of Ben Brusey and everyone at Penguin Random House. They provided the platform for this book and helped me in so many ways. It has been a pleasure working with Ben and the team: Rebecca Ikin, Olivia Thomas, Penny Liechti, Jessica Fletcher, Laurie Ip Fung Chun, Anna Cowling, Emma Grey Gelder, Alice Gomer, Kirsten Greenwood, Jade Unwin, Lewis Cain, Emily Harvey, Phoenix Curland, Meredith Benson.

I was initially overwhelmed when Don McRae said he would work with me. I always remember the first-ever interview Rob and I did with Don, back in May 2021, and that encouraged me to approach him with the idea of our collaborating together. Thank you, Don, for creating a beautiful memoir. Your talent and love of writing shines through and I look forward to sharing the book with my children, and their children, in many years to come. It has been an honour and a privilege to co-write this book with you and thanks again for your patience and your kindness. The writing of *Take Care* was a team effort and we worked so well together.

Special thanks to Prince William for writing the foreword. Your heartfelt words mean so much to me and all the family. Rob would have been very proud.

Rob's former teammates, Barrie McDermott and Kevin Sinfield helped so much, and their memories and insights made a great contribution to the book. Thanks, also, to my friend Angela for always being there for me and helping me piece all the memories together from over the years. So much thanks to all of you. Without your generous contributions, this book would not have been possible.

Thank you also to:

My employer, Leeds Teaching Hospitals NHS Trust, and colleagues within the NHS, for being so supportive.

To the Leeds Hospitals Charity, which I am a proud patron of, for supporting the specialist MND care centre appeal. The centre will be a legacy to Rob and will provide patients and their families with the best possible care.

A heartfelt and massive thank you to our amazing NHS staff who provided extraordinary care for Rob throughout his illness. You made our journey with MND as good as it could be. I can never repay you for the care and compassion that you showed our family, but I hope you know how truly grateful I am.

I want to pay tribute to all the unpaid carers who selflessly dedicate their time and energy to caring for their loved ones. Your compassion and sacrifice do not go unnoticed. You are the unsung heroes who embody strength, resilience and unconditional love.

Thank you to everyone in my wonderful family, especially my mum and dad, who go above and beyond for me and the children every single day. Your unwavering love and support means the world.

I want to say a really huge thank you to our children, Macy, Maya and Jackson. You have been my tower of strength. You give me a reason to smile every day. I am so proud of you. I love you all so very much.

Finally, thank you Rob, for choosing me to be your wife. I couldn't have wished for a better husband and father to our three children. I miss you every single day. You taught us how to live each day to its fullest and I am determined to make you proud. I love you with all my heart x

Credits

Photography credits

p. 5, top left and right images: Copyright © BBC Breakfast
p. 6, bottom right image: Copyright © Charlie Mackesy 2023

The author and publisher gratefully acknowledge the permission granted to reproduce the above copyright material in this book.

Text acknowledgements

p. 40: Lines from 'Peggy Sue', recorded by Buddy Holly (1957); written by Buddy Holly, Jerry Allison and Norman Petty. Lyrics © Mpl Music Publishing Inc, BMG Gold Songs and Mpl Music Publishing, Inc. o/b/o Wren Music Co.

pp. 101 and 275: Lines taken from the film *Any Given Sunday*. Screenplay co-written by William Oliver Stone and John Logan. Directed by William Oliver Stone, Final Cut, Warner Bros. 1999